DV to DIVA

L J Kulow

DV to DIVA

CONTENTS

DEDICATION viii

INTRODUCTION 1
BEFORE YOU BEGIN 4
WELCOME 9
PART ONE – I AM DIVINE 13
Part one tools & practices 37
PART TWO – I AM INTELLIGENT 43
Part two tools & practices 66
PART THREE – I AM VIBRANT 73
Part three tools & practices 95
Part 4 – I AM AUTHENIC 103
Part four tools & practices 132
THE END? 141
THE CYCLE OF VIOLENCE 145
ADDITIONAL INFORMATION 150

- EMOTIONAL FREEDOM TECHNIQUE 165
- ADDITIONAL TOOLS & PRACTICES 188
- Crisis Support Resources 199

Copyright © 2025 by L J Kulow
All rights reserved. No part of this book may be reproduced in any manner whatsoever without written permission except in the case of brief quotations embodied in critical articles and reviews.
First Printing, 2025

Dedication

This book is dedicated to you, yes you—reading these words right now and to all who walk with the pain of a DV experience. We have the power to break the cycles, to make the invisible, visible, to transform the story, and to create a world of healing and hope for ourselves and others. Your journey from DV to DIVA inspires us all. Thank you for being here, thank you for being you.

INTRODUCTION

DIVA – Divine, Intelligent, Vibrant, Authentic.

Written by a DIVA who's been there, a woman who has lived through domestic violence and risen up from it, this transformational guide offers hope and healing to women rebuilding their lives after DV.

DV to DIVA isn't just a story of survival, it's about how we can all thrive as the Divine, Intelligent, Vibrant and Authentic women we were always meant to be. It's about empowerment, inspiration and possibility. It's about moving beyond the shadows of abuse to embrace our true value.

This book is a celebration of resilience and transformation. It addresses the unique challenges we face as domestic violence 'survivors' while providing actionable strategies for creating lasting change. Through practical tools and proven techniques, we'll explore the powerful connection between body, mind, and soul, learning to heal holistically from the inside out. These pages offer insights, encouragement, inspiration and practical wisdom from lived experience.

Whether you're just beginning your healing journey or ready to step fully into your power, *DV to DIVA* reminds you that your past does not define your future. You are not broken. You are a beautiful woman with unlimited potential. It's time to reclaim yourself and live the empowered, authentic life you deserve.

How to Use This Book

This book is your companion on the journey from DV to DIVA. It has been carefully structured to guide you through reclaiming yourself including your spirit, your mind, your vitality, and your authentic self.

DV to DIVA is organized into four main interconnected parts, each representing a facet of the woman you are becoming. While designed to be read part by part from beginning to end, these sections are deeply interwoven. You'll notice themes and concepts introduced in one part that are explored more deeply in another. As you progress through each part, you'll build layers of understanding, with each section informing and enriching the others.

These four parts don't exist in silos—they dance together, support one another, and collectively work to create the whole, empowered you. You may find yourself returning to earlier parts with fresh eyes and discovering new meaning as your journey unfolds. The healing journey is rarely linear, and this book is designed to meet you wherever you are as you grow.

Part 1. Divine; goddess like. Reconnecting with our spiritual self.

Part 2. Intelligent; acquiring and applying knowledge and skills. Trusting our intuition and rebuilding confidence in our decisions.

Part 3. Vibrant; full of life and energy. Restoring our physical and mental health and embracing joyful living.

Part 4. Authentic; genuine and true to self. Honouring our inner voice and desires without fear or apology.

Additional sections at the end of part four provide practical resources, deeper insights and more tools and techniques to support your ongoing journey, offering practices you can return to again and again as you continue to grow into your power. Remember: You are not broken. You are becoming. And you are already divine, intelligent, vibrant, and authentic—this book simply helps you remember what was always within you.

BEFORE YOU BEGIN

IMPORTANT: Please read before beginning your *DV to DIVA* journey.

This book is designed for the journey after domestic violence.

If you are currently living with DV, your immediate safety is the most important thing. Please see the resources page at the back of this book for a list of resources in Australia.

There may be a voice in your mind telling you that today was better, that it will be okay, that things will change and so you stay. I understand that voice—I lived with it for too long. From my experience, and from what countless other 'survivors' and professionals have shared, domestic violence does not get better on its own. It does not change. The pattern continues, the cycle continues, and often escalates. There is information explaining the cycle of violence on *Page 145* of this book.

I stayed in a dangerous environment longer than I should have. I was terrified of what might happen if I left, and there were days I thought everything was getting better and the worst was over. My mind had literally been reprogrammed over the years. The perpetrator I lived with used threats and manipulation as chains to keep me trapped, "If you leave, I will find you and kill you" and "If you leave, I'll end my life and it will be your fault" and "If you leave, how will you manage on your own?—you need me".

There were many more threats, each one designed to hold me in a place of fear and control. There were also emotional tactics, reminding me we were soul mates, meant to be, life partners. He would sob saying he couldn't live without me and ask, "How could you ruin this, ruin us?" before turning it on me with comments like "You just want to control me". It's frightening and confusing at the same time.

None of these sayings were true. All of them were manipulation.

The Truth About Leaving

I needed to because I was at the point where I was certain he would end my life, either accidently or deliberately. Yes, it was difficult—incredibly, devastatingly difficult. But that difficult journey became the beginning of me finding my path again and living a better life. The threats that seemed so real, so terrifying, turned out to be empty words designed to keep me small and scared.

You are stronger than you know. You are more capable than you've been allowed to believe. You deserve safety, respect, and love—real love, not the twisted version that comes wrapped in violence and control. You are not alone. There are many supports available to help you leave safely and rebuild your life.

A New Life, A Newer Version of You

As you embark on this new chapter of life with the *DV to DIVA* book and accompanying materials and courses, please be aware that the content may contain triggering material related to domestic violence experiences. This is a natural part of the healing and transformation process.

Please Remember:

- Continue using your existing support systems - Keep in regular contact with your counsellors, therapists, support groups, and other health professionals.
- This book is a tool based on my lived experience and opinions and is not a replacement for professional practice. These materials are designed to assist and complement your healing journey and is not a substitute for professional mental health care.
- Honor your pace - If you encounter triggering content, take breaks as needed and reach out for support. There is also an exercise on *Page 96* to assist.
- Your safety comes first . If you are in an unsafe situation, please prioritize your immediate safety and contact appropriate emergency services or domestic violence supports.

Please refer to the *Resources* page at the back of this book for additional support.

What to Expect

Much of this book focuses on energy and vibration. After all, everything in the universe, including your physical body, your thoughts, and the environment around you, is energy!

The perspectives and approaches shared in this book are drawn from my lived experience, extensive personal research, and what has worked for me and many others. While I've endeavoured to share evidence-based practices where possible, some content reflects my personal opinions and interpretations formed through my healing journey. This book is designed as a starting point and is not comprehensive in any area. I hope it will inspire you to gently explore more of the world around you to find new ways of being and to find your path.

If you read something that really gets under your skin or agitates you, please stay with it. Don't let discomfort become a reason to close the book or give up. The friction you're feeling is often pointing to something important. Use it as a clue to explore what's happening for you, there are techniques about this later in the book.

There may be tools and techniques in this book that are completely new for you. These techniques work! And not just for me but for thousands of people around the globe who use them.

While there is no quick fix to anything in life, and while the techniques and information I share will create incredible life transformation, sometimes much sooner than expected, don't put a time limit on yourself. Practice the techniques, each practice is like strengthening muscles. Do a little each day. Don't underestimate the power of one small action. You got this.

WELCOME

Affirm now.

I am Divine. I am Goddess like.

I am Intelligent. I am acquiring and applying knowledge and skills.

I am Vibrant. I am full of life and energy.

I am Authentic. I am genuine and true to self.

I am all of the above and I am a woman who lived with DV. I've been there. So I know, to say these words is almost instantly jarring and feels not at all true. I didn't feel goddess like, I felt broken, exhausted and ashamed. I didn't feel intelligent at all, I felt stupid and small. I didn't feel vibrant, I felt sick and weak. And authentic was simply a word that had no meaning to me.

But there was a little part of me, maybe it was anger, maybe something else, that refused to accept this as my defining experience. That little part whispered as though through clenched teeth, "I won't let this break me!"

My journey through domestic violence and out the other side was long, painful, heartbreaking and difficult. When I applied for a domestic violence protection order (DVO), the magistrate described the case as one of the worst they had seen.

After finally leaving the relationship, which alone took many attempts, I spent a decade on a journey to find myself, my hope, my dreams, and my joy. I spent years of trying different techniques and time crying when it seemed they didn't work. Years of trying to be normal, trying not to be broken. I kept trying and trying, feeling like I was never getting anywhere, never achieving anything. Nothing I was trying was working.

I studied myself. I studied energy. I studied anything I thought might help me get from a life of despair to a life of feeling like a DIVA—feeling like my true self again.

I stumbled. I fell. I lost hope. I was triggered. I was angry. I was hurting. I was alone. It was a long journey.

At times it felt absolutely impossible. Everything good seemed out of reach, made for someone else. There was nothing empowering in my life. There were days I just wanted to lay on the grass and melt into the earth. I didn't want to play anymore. Life was horrible, one hard day after another.

I couldn't see a future for myself. I was just getting through day by day, one step at a time. My mind had been so programmed to believe I was worthless and useless that I honestly thought my life would just go on being one of simple survival, just getting by on a tiny budget, maybe on a government benefit, with no abilities, independence or strength of my own. I felt totally disabled and like I had failed life and life had failed me.

I was heartbroken and broken but there had to be more, and I wanted more. I questioned life. Why is life so awful? Why are people so nasty? What is life even about? Why am I here? Why did this happen to me?

I wanted to feel good. I wanted to feel happy. I wanted to feel alive. I wanted to live, and not just be alive, but live, like other people do. I hated feeling rubbish and I hated my feelings.

Today, I do feel good, better than good! I feel alive again! But it took years of healing for me. Years of searching for knowledge, study and practice to get to where I am today. It took tears and hope. It took delving into moments of pain, feeling utterly alone, lost, helpless and beaten to rediscover my true self and become me again.

I never had someone who truly understood, someone who had walked this path before me and could say, "I know. I've been there too". I stumbled through my healing alone, searching desperately for answers, wishing someone would just show me the way.

That's why I'm here now—to be the support I never had. To share the tools I wish someone had given me years ago, so your healing doesn't have to drag on the way mine did. You don't have to figure this out alone. You don't have to spend a decade searching in the dark.

I've lived this experience and I've found my way through. Now I want to walk alongside you, sharing what I've learned—practical, lifelong tools that can help you reclaim yourself and build the life you deserve, much sooner than I did.

I am not a licensed health professional, but I hold an associate degree in Applied Social Science and am an accredited EFT Practitioner. The content in this book draws from my lived experience with domestic violence and my journey of study, healing and using various techniques to regain quality of life. It's a roller coaster of ups and downs, but you got this. You are ok, you are stronger than you know.

I have written this book specifically for women survivors of domestic violence. Although I respectfully acknowledge everyone who has experienced DV regardless of gender, the reality is that we as women are the majority who experience severe and repeated violence from intimate partners. This book honours our reality.

Let's go DIVA and embark on this transformative journey together. From damaged to Divine. From incapacitated to Intelligent. From victim to Vibrant. From assaulted to Authentic.

PART ONE – I AM DIVINE

Reconnecting with our spiritual self.

When I speak of your divine nature, I'm talking about the essence of who you are beyond all the labels, roles, and stories you've been told about yourself or that you have created about yourself. This is the part of you that existed before anyone ever made you feel small, before anyone ever questioned your worth, before any trauma touched your spirit. Your divine self is the pure consciousness that flows through you—the spark of infinite possibility that connects you to something greater than yourself. It's your intuition, your innate wisdom, your capacity for unconditional love, and your natural ability to create, transform and expand. It is important to know from the very beginning, you are not a body. You are divine energy having a physical experience. You are the vibration of pure love, you are energy.

Energy and Vibration: The Foundation of Everything

Everything in our universe is energy. All energy is vibration of varying frequencies. Our thoughts, emotions, our bodies, the things around us—all exist as energetic patterns that resonate and interact with the environment we live in. Understanding this energetic nature of existence provides insight into how we develop our sense of self-love and self-worth, and how we can become trapped in destructive patterns or relationships.

As babies, we entered this world already loving ourselves, knowing our pure connection to the universe and recognizing our inherent divinity. In fact, we are not connected to the universe but simply and energetically a part of it. In those early moments after birth, our energetic vibration was pure, unfiltered, and naturally aligned with love and self-acceptance. We didn't question our worth or wonder if we deserved care and affection—we simply existed in a state of being that naturally attracted what we needed.

This initial state represents our truest energetic vibration: one of unconditional self-love, openness, and infinite possibility. Before language, before concepts of "good" and "bad", before the complex web of social conditioning began to take hold, we vibrated at the frequency of pure potential.

As we develop, the programming from our parents, family members, friends, teachers, and society begins to shape our energetic signature. We are raised on the vibrations around us, absorbing the emotional frequencies of our environment like energetic sponges. Every interaction, every spoken word, every unspoken tension or moment of joy becomes part of our developing energetic blueprint.

We form our beliefs and perceptions from the energies around us—not just from what people tell us, but from the vibrational quality of how they treat us, how they treat themselves, and how they move through the world. A parent's encouragement becomes a familiar frequency of "I can do this", while constant criticism becomes a frequency of "not enough".

Over time, these external influences begin to shift our natural vibration. If we're surrounded by love, acceptance, and healthy boundaries, our energetic frequency tends to remain relatively high, maintaining much of that original self-love and connection to our inherent worth. However, if we're exposed to criticism, neglect, abuse, or emotional instability, our vibration gradually adjusts to match these lower frequencies.

How Control Patterns Develop

Everyone experiences this conditioning, including those who eventually become perpetrators of domestic violence. They too were once babies who entered the world with that pure, loving vibration. They too absorbed the energetic patterns of their environment, often learning early on that certain behaviours—tantrums, manipulation, emotional outbursts—could get them what they needed. A child wanting attention from a parent, demanding a toy, or refusing to eat learns quickly: control works.

When these patterns continue unchecked into adulthood, they become a deeply ingrained way of meeting needs and managing anxiety. The vibration shifts from "I am safe and loved" to "I must control to survive".

These control-based vibrations often develop in environments where fear rather than trust, is the primary tool for managing behaviour. Parents operating from their own unhealed patterns may use control not from malice, but because it's the only frequency they know. They genuinely love their children and want the best for them, but having absorbed similar energies from their own upbringing, they unconsciously pass on a vibration where control equals safety and love must be earned through compliance.

Many of us have learned to comply through fear—it's not just a family pattern, it's woven into the fabric of society itself. "Pay the fine or else", "Follow the rules or face consequences", "Do as you're told or suffer the punishment". Fear-based control is so normalized that we often don't even recognize it as such. We've been conditioned to respond to threats, to avoid consequences, to keep our heads down and comply. This makes fear a familiar frequency, one that feels almost... normal.

Perpetrators of domestic violence adopt and perfect this same fear-based method of controlling. They've learned it works—in childhood, in society, in every system around them. They simply apply it with precision to their intimate relationships, using the threat of consequences (anger, withdrawal, violence, abandonment) to ensure compliance and maintain their sense of control.

It's important to understand this isn't about blaming parents or pointing fingers at anyone's upbringing. All parents are doing their absolute best with the emotional tools they have. Society itself reinforces these patterns through cultural messages about power, gender roles, and what it means to be "strong" or "in charge". The energy of control is woven through generations, through media, through institutions—it becomes a familiar frequency that feels normal even when it's harmful.

Mental health issues can certainly amplify these patterns, but at the core, domestic violence is fundamentally about control—and that control is rooted in learned vibrational patterns that say "I am only safe when I am in charge of everything and everyone around me".

How Domestic Violence Traps Your Energy

So, what happens when someone vibrating at this frequency of control encounters someone vibrating at a frequency of gentleness, kindness, and empathy?

Perpetrators of domestic violence are often highly attuned to energy, even if they wouldn't describe it that way. They unconsciously seek out partners whose vibrational patterns make them particularly vulnerable to manipulation—people who are naturally giving, who want to see the good in others, who have been conditioned to prioritize others' needs over their own.

The perpetrator begins to systematically undermine everything that is essentially you. They chip away at your sense of self-worth using calculated tactics that happen so gradually you don't even realize it's happening. Your vibration—once aligned with self-love and possibility—starts to shift. You begin to resonate with their frequency: "not good enough", "too sensitive", "the problem".

This is how domestic violence exploits your energy. The perpetrator has spent a lifetime tuning their behaviour to maintain complete control over their environment, which includes the people in it. They've learned that when they feel anxious, uncertain, or threatened, they can restore their sense of safety by controlling you—your thoughts, your movements, your emotions, your very sense of reality.

And because you're an energetic being absorbing the vibrations around you, just as you did as a child, you begin to match this lower frequency. The voice that once whispered "you deserve better" gets quieter and quieter, drowned out by the constant hum of "you're not enough" that now fills your energetic space.

It might start with love-bombing, showering you with attention and affection to draw you in. Over time they slowly introduce criticism disguised as concern or help. They'll isolate you from friends and family, making you more dependent on them for validation. They control the finances, so you literally become financially dependent on them. They gaslight you (I had never heard this term before!) making you question your own memory and perception of reality until you start doubting yourself constantly and begin thinking you are crazy. Then they begin using threats and intimidation as manipulative tactics to keep you under their control, and they know exactly which emotional buttons to press to keep you feeling small and walking on eggshells.

This is not your fault. You didn't create this situation. You simply encountered a vibrational pattern more powerful and more practiced than your own awareness at that time. Understanding this is the first step toward reclaiming your true frequency—the one you were born with, the one that knows your divine worth.

You deserve better. You deserve love, confidence, peace and happiness. At the point of becoming involved with a perpetrator of DV, there was already some programming in you, some thought or belief that you are not good enough—and that's our starting point. They didn't create your vulnerability, they didn't make you crazy, they simply recognized an opportunity and exploited your kindness, gentleness and yes, I'll say it, your weakness. The reason they do this, the reason they have a desperate need to have control, is primarily because of their own lack of self-worth and their own disconnect from their divinity.

My Self-worth journey

I had sailed through life with no real plans. I was earning good money as a single woman with solid jobs, and later started work in the financial sector. I had investments, cash and debts. My life became boozy lunches with people who loved them just as much as I did. Lavish weekends away at expensive hotels and resorts, flights to here and there and I wore expensive clothes and jewellery. I was always showing off my wealth and my wit. I felt good. I felt confident. I thought I was happy.

But it was all a false sense of self. I didn't know who I really was, and back then, it didn't even cross my mind to want to know.

The day my life trajectory changed was after a visit to the doctor. By then I had sold off the investments, paid off most of my debts and had accumulated a saving for a deposit on a property. Even though I was still working in finance, I was living fortnightly pay to fortnightly pay. The lavish lunches were long gone. I wasn't living that loud, fancy life anymore. I'd settled down. It was just me and my dog (a gorgeous, fabulous big dog, by the way!) in a quieter, calmer life. I was content and happy doing my thing.

One day, I caught the flu and had it for long enough that I was frustrated enough to go to the doctor. He looked at me and asked two questions. "Why are you not married? You are beautiful, you are generally healthy, but you live with your dog! What are you doing with your life?". At the time, I laughed his comments off, took my script for some flu meds and left. But the questions ate away at me, and I realized my feeling of content was shallow and the confidence I showed on the outside was skin deep. I unconsciously felt a sense of "I am not enough".

The subconscious beliefs brought to the surface that day was, I was nothing. I was not enough and not worthy. My life wasn't good enough. I wasn't ok just being me. And while the "not good enough" ran deeper than just having a partner, in that doctor's eyes, being chosen by a man was what gave me worth. It was the proof I needed that I mattered, that I was visible, that I had value. My worth wasn't a given—it was something bestowed upon me only when and if a man decided I was worthy of his attention. Without that validation, without that choice, I was somehow incomplete.

This isn't new—it's an ancient script we've been handed down. Historically, women were treated as items to be selected, their worth determined by dowries their families offered to sweeten the deal. We were commodities on a market, our value artificially inflated or diminished based on what we brought to a transaction. And while we've come so far, that ancient belief still lurks beneath seemingly innocent questions: "Why aren't you married yet?". As if marriage is the measure of a woman's success. As if a woman standing alone, building her life, healing from trauma, isn't already whole. As if we need to be chosen to be worthy. But here's the truth: You don't become valuable because someone chooses you. You are valuable because you exist. You are worthy because you are here, breathing, surviving, rising. No man—no person—has the power to grant or revoke that worth. It was always yours.

None of this had come into my conscious thoughts at the time, so, when I met a very charming man at a volunteer function one evening, it seemed that things were on the up for me. He seemed charming and attentive, he was tall, dark and handsome in that classic way that made other women glance twice. His attention felt intoxicating after a period of time being single. At the time I wasn't looking for a relationship and it took me by surprise—I was swept off my feet in this new romance. I remember other women commenting to me how lucky I was and that I deserved to be happy.

He remembered every detail I shared, asked thoughtful questions, and seemed completely interested in me. He made me feel like I was the only person in the room when we were together. For those first few weeks, I felt seen and valued in ways I hadn't experienced before. The flowers arrived, the compliments flowed freely, and he seemed genuinely interested in me and my dreams.

When I reflect on this now, I see it clearly: he was interviewing me. In fact, he had placed himself at the volunteer function that night with one intention, to find someone like me. Every question he asked was designed to gauge what kind of person I was, to map my vulnerabilities, to determine if I was a match for his control. He was gathering intelligence—learning my weak spots, my insecurities, my desires—so he could position himself as exactly what I wanted and needed.

I didn't notice how quickly he wanted to spend every evening together, or that within months we were living together. I didn't notice how he subtly discouraged my girls' nights out, or how his loving concern about my "toxic" friendships gradually isolated me from most of my friends. He even had me believing my family were unsupportive, and I became isolated from them too. But when someone makes you feel like you're floating, it's easy to mistake the ground disappearing beneath your feet for simply soaring higher.

In reality, I had ended up in an extremely dangerous DV situation that got to the point where I was terrified. I thought I was "the crazy one" and the violence became so bad that I believed I would lose my life. I was at rock bottom, and I know you know where that is.

Leaving him became a cycle of failed attempts, each one ending with me staying in the relationship, convinced by his careful conditioning that I lacked the strength, resources, or capability to have a life without him, or that he would end his own life if I did leave, and I would be responsible for it. I had never heard of the "Cycle of DV" but I was deeply in it. He had convinced me that I was the cause of his going from charming gentleman to violent beast. One night came with such violence and terror that I did not believe I would see the light of the next morning. I locked myself in a room, terrified to leave out of the window because I knew if he heard it open, he would instantly be there on the outside. I had given up and accepted my fate. I fell asleep on the cold timber floor, praying and utterly exhausted.

To my surprise I woke the next morning, sore and tired and from there, I began a new journey, one that took me years to get back on my feet. I felt like I had come out of the frying pan, into the fire—a saying that I had heard once when I was a child. I thought life would be better when I left, but it was just as difficult. Over the years he had spent all of my savings and not only that, had raised thousands of dollars of debts in my name that I didn't know about. On top of everything else I was experiencing; I was financially devastated, starting again with nothing.

I shakily bumped my way through life feeling desperate and depleted. I was trying all the success programs, three steps to this and five steps to that, reading self-help books, registering for masterclasses and nothing seemed to have the results I expected or needed. Does this sound familiar?

In hindsight now, I wasn't looking at the "wrong" things—I just didn't have them in the right order. I also needed to learn more about energy, thoughts and the human body before I could build the solid foundation my life stands on now.

The Mirror of Self-Worth

When I started to look at myself and check in with my own self-worth, the shocking realization hit me: the perpetrator I was involved with was a mirror of how I saw myself. He had tapped into my unconscious beliefs about myself. Beliefs I didn't know I had, beliefs of "I am not worthy."

When I looked back at how those beliefs and patterns came to be there, it started to make sense. I could not possibly have had the experiences of someone who loved and respected themselves, because my subconscious programming was that of "I am not worthy."

There is a quote that is perhaps a paraphrase of the writings of Carl Jung, and it goes something like this: until you make the unconscious conscious, it will direct your life. In other words, our unconscious programming, or our subconscious programming, is what is running the show of life. I had become consciously aware that some of my subconscious beliefs and patterns were rooted in the idea that I was not worthy. So where did this programming come from?

I can't remember how I saw the world as a kid, but I didn't always feel safe. I was never seen as a bright kid, often told to focus or stop daydreaming. I was not "switched on" and although I loved to read, I failed nearly every test I did in primary school.

I showed my teacher my test results one day after not getting a single answer correct and she brushed me away saying, "You must be stupid then". I remember standing there, fixed in that moment of time as those words deeply sank in.

My parents raised me to be prepared to live in a world that was cruel, full of overseas wars, local crimes, violence, teenage pregnancies and AIDS. They wanted me to be strong and capable of living in such a world, but it seemed their only vision for me was a despaired prediction of me living in the slums, barefoot and pregnant. Compounded maybe, by my proven inability to learn anything. I would amount to nothing. At the same time, I was raised to be kind, considerate, polite and respectful to others. I had developed beliefs that I was stupid and that I would amount to nothing. These beliefs were the source of my lack of self-worth.

It makes sense then, that when I met a perpetrator of DV, the love bombing and charm, the attention and affection, felt like everything I'd ever wanted and never had. It was proof—finally—that I was worthy and loveable. There I was, important in a relationship. I thought someone loved me for who I was.

For a while I'd buried those thoughts and feelings of lack of self-worth. I'd convinced myself I was happy and smart. After all, I'd bought investments, I was earning good money, I was holding down solid job roles, and now I was building a life with someone.

And for a while, life seemed good. But DV slowly and surely took hold.

Through the process of living with domestic violence, those old beliefs came roaring back to the surface. "I am stupid". "I am unworthy". They'd been there all along, just waiting.

What I didn't know then was that beneath all those false beliefs, something else had been there all along, something true remained... and that was my divine nature.

Your Divine Essence is Untouchable

There's a spiritual truth that I discovered and that is: no matter what has been done to us, no matter how broken we feel, there is something within us that remains untouchable, undamaged, and absolutely sacred. It is our divine self—the part of the universe that vibrates as pure love. Call it our soul, our essence, our divine spark, our inner light—the name doesn't matter. It was an absolute comfort to know there was a part of me that wasn't hurt and broken, even if I didn't feel like I had immediate access to it.

What matters is understanding that this part of us exists beyond the reach of any abuser, any trauma, any circumstance. It's the part of us that is connected to something greater even in our darkest moments. We are energetically a part of this great universe. We are the Divine and we have a body. Our body lives in us and we are having this human experience. So, I am, and you are Divine.

I know this might be hard to believe, especially if you feel shattered, if you look in the mirror and don't recognize the person staring back, if you feel like the abuse changed you at your very core. The pain is real, the damage to your sense of self is real, but underneath all of that, your divine essence remains intact. You are okay. I know this.

Think of it like this: Picture the sun, a beautiful, brilliant light covered by layers of cloud. The cloud doesn't change the nature of the sun, it just obscures it. The abuse, the trauma, the years of being told you were worthless—these are the clouds. But the sun itself—you!—that's eternal, that's unbreakable, that's you.

Also, think of it like this: you hold a puppy in your arms. You love this puppy. Your heart glows when you hold him. This divine being matters and is loveable. Not because of what he does, not because of how useful he might be to others, not because he is "good enough", but because he exists. This is the same for you. Your Divine being matters and is loveable. Not because of what you do, not because of how useful you might be to others, not because you are "good enough", but because you exist. You are the same energy as the puppy! Loveable, beautiful, unique.

Some days, connecting back to this truth feels impossible. I know. Some days, the cloud feels so thick you can't imagine there's any light underneath. That's okay. The sun doesn't need your belief to keep shining. It doesn't need your permission to be sacred. It simply is, and so are you.

When we begin to truly understand this—not just intellectually, but in our subconscious—everything changes. We stop looking to others to determine our worth because we realize our worth was always there. We stop accepting being treated in ways that don't honour the sacred beings that we are. We start making choices from love rather than fear, because we remember that love is our true nature.

The journey back to ourselves is really a journey back to this knowing of our divinity. It's about clearing away the clouds, healing the wounds, and remembering who we've always been underneath it all: sacred, worthy, powerful beings of light who deserve nothing less than the best life has to offer, especially from ourselves.

Understanding Self-Worth as Vibrational Frequency

Lack of self-worth is a disconnect from our true divinity—a separation from source, from our roots, from our authentic self. Our level of self-worth is essentially our energetic frequency, how we vibrate in relationship to ourselves and the world. When our self-worth is high, we naturally vibrate at frequencies that attract respect, love, and healthy relationships, and we can live from a place of knowing our divinity. When our self-worth is low, we vibrate at frequencies that may attract or tolerate disrespect, manipulation, or abuse.

This energetic principle explains why simply telling someone to "love themselves more" or "know their worth" often isn't enough to create lasting change. To shift our self-worth, we must actually shift our vibrational frequency, and this requires more than just changing our thoughts. It involves healing the energetic wounds that keep us vibrating at lower frequencies and consciously choosing to align with higher vibrational states.

I had no idea where to start with aligning with higher vibrational states, so I began to study more of this. The main message for me in those early studies was that there was no way for me to instantaneously shift from a low vibration into a higher one. It needed to be a step-by-step process, and it required small (but powerful) changes in my behaviours and habits. Initially, I thought the smallest change would only create the smallest result—but that's not how it works. The smallest change is actually an energetic change in direction, a change in vibration, and this new frequency creates noticeable results. The new frequency paves the way for more new frequencies and so the vibrational shift is activated. The analogy of a compass changing one point in direction really resonated with me.

Imagine you're bush walking with a compass, and your compass is off true North by just one point. If you keep walking in that slightly wrong direction, you'll end up kilometres away from your intended destination. However, if you adjust it back to true North—just that tiny correction—you'll arrive at your intended place. Any small adjustment in direction changes your entire journey.

The same principle applies to raising your vibration. A small shift in your energetic frequency, like adjusting a compass by one point, can completely transform the direction of your life experience. We are divine vibrational beings. Sometimes life circumstances pull us into lower vibrational states, but we always have the ability to take the path back to our true vibrational nature.

The journey back to our authentic vibrational frequency is both deeply personal and universally healing. As we raise our own vibration, we not only transform our own lives but contribute to the healing of the collective energetic field, making it easier for others to access their own higher frequencies and break free from cycles of harm and disconnection.

But here's where many of us get stuck: we understand that we need to shift our vibration, we know we need to change our frequency, yet we can't seem to make it happen. We try affirmations, we read the books, we attend the workshops—and still, that inner voice keeps whispering "not worthy", "not good enough", "not lovable". Why? Because our conscious mind might understand we deserve better, but our subconscious mind is still running the old program. The beliefs formed during our earliest years, reinforced through trauma and abuse, have become deeply embedded patterns operating beneath our awareness.

Understanding the Whole of You

I have always believed that the body, mind and soul, for want of better descriptive words, are not just connected but pieces of the whole that is us for this human experience. Healthy mind, healthy body. The soul that utilizes them whilst having this human experience is eternal and connected for this lifetime experience. We are souls, our bodies are in our souls (not the other way around—we are not souls stuck in our bodies) and we are having a human experience, experiencing all the senses that only a physical body can have. The divine nature of us is love and we can extend that love to our bodies, our minds, our environment and everything and everyone in it.

Self-love is an essential recognition of the divine essence that is us. When we truly love ourselves, we acknowledge that we are spiritual beings having a human experience, worthy of love not because of what we do, but because of who we are at our core. This spiritual self-love means honouring the soul that chose this particular journey, with all its lessons, challenges, and growth opportunities.

The DV Experience as Growth

Yes! This experience we have just had, our brush with DV, was an experience and it is really helpful to see it as such. It's difficult to do at first, I'll admit that, but through the exercises I'll share with you, this concept gets easier. Not only is it an experience, but it is also a growth opportunity. Not in the sense of those annoying little sayings, "What doesn't kill us makes us stronger", and such, but in the sense of asking, "What's possible here? How can I grow from this? What's good about this? What is the blessing in this?".

When these questions are asked, the universe delivers the answers and new perspectives arrive. Seeing the experience from a different perspective is expansive. But this all needs to come from a place of compassion, not judgment. We cannot judge ourselves for being in this experience, but ultimately, it's how we use the experience to grow. Having compassion and developing greater self-love will allow space for this growth.

When we embrace self-love from this divine perspective, we stop seeing ourselves as broken beings needing to be fixed and start recognizing ourselves as perfect souls learning and expanding through this human experience. This spiritual foundation of self-acceptance creates an unshakeable inner sanctuary, a place of inner peace that external circumstances cannot disturb. And so here is the beginning of changing the vibration. Your vibration, once in this space, will never again be in alignment with lower vibrations of experiences like DV.

From this space of divine self-love, we naturally extend authentic compassion to others, knowing that we are all interconnected souls supporting each other's growth. Self-love becomes not just personal healing, but a contribution to the collective awakening of humanity. What if everyone loved themselves this much?

Self-worth - The Foundation of Everything

Self-love/self-worth allows us to recognize our inherent worth, independent of our achievements, relationships, or perceived mistakes. It allows us to set boundaries that protect our wellbeing, to pursue goals that align with our values rather than seeking validation from others, and to recover from setbacks without falling into destructive self-criticism. Without self-love, we become vulnerable to toxic relationships, burnout, and the exhausting cycle of trying to earn our worth through external approval.

When we genuinely love ourselves, we make decisions from a place of strength rather than fear, we attract healthier relationships because we model how we deserve to be treated, and we develop the resilience to weather life's inevitable challenges. Self-love is the difference between surviving and thriving.

But I wasn't there yet. Not even close.

The divine future self – releasing the victim mindset

I was unable to see myself as a strong, powerful, beautiful woman—comfortable in my own skin, confident and safe. I was unable to feel my divinity; in fact, I didn't identify myself as a divine being at all. I thought I was simply a human body that someone had hurt. I had no ability to switch my thoughts from where they were to where they are now. I was trapped in a cage of my own limiting beliefs, unable to see beyond the identity of someone who had been broken.

From a vibrational perspective, remember, it is not possible to move instantaneously from a lower vibration to a higher one. And where I was vibrating at that time was the frequency of victimhood—one of the lowest frequencies we can inhabit. It's a frequency of powerlessness, of things happening to us rather than for us or through us. When we're vibrating as a victim, we unconsciously broadcast "I am helpless, I am broken, I am defined by what was done to me". This vibration becomes our identity, our story, our energetic signature—and it keeps us trapped in patterns that reinforce that very belief.

I lived in this vibration for years without even realizing it. The victim mindset had woven itself so deeply into my sense of self that I couldn't imagine existing without it. It was in how I introduced myself, how I explained my circumstances, how I related to others. It became my identity.

Then one day, I heard the words fall out of my mouth that had been holding me in that persona for years: "Well, I've come out of DV and..."

It was a gut-wrenching moment.

In that instant, I realized I was still identifying myself through the lens of what had happened to me. I was still wearing the victim story like a badge, still vibrating at that frequency of "wounded woman". And as long as I held that identity, I could never truly step into my power. I could never see myself as the divine, strong, capable woman I was meant to become.

This is the challenge so many of us face: we've been conditioned to believe that acknowledging our suffering, naming our trauma, and identifying as survivors means we must continue to define ourselves by what was done to us. Even labelling myself as a "survivor" kept me at a certain vibrational level—it was a step up from victim, yes, a higher rung on the ladder, but it still defined me by what I had survived rather than who I was becoming.

But there's a profound difference between acknowledging your past and allowing it to define your present and future.

Releasing the victim mindset doesn't mean denying what happened or pretending the pain wasn't real. It means shifting your vibrational identity from "I am someone this happened to" to "I am someone who is moving through this toward something greater".

You will need to let go of all the stories associated with being broken and not good enough, especially the victim story that may have become deeply embedded in your identity.

While this victim narrative once served as a survival mechanism—helping you navigate an impossible situation—you don't need that protective story anymore. The reasons you developed attachment to this role don't matter now because they were simply survival instincts doing their job. Now it's time to release that old identity and step into not just who you're truly meant to be, but who you truly are.

Your future self—your divine self—already exists at a higher vibrational frequency. She is strong, powerful, confident, and free. She knows her worth. She moves through the world with grace and certainty. She is not defined by her past but empowered by her journey through it. Having the ability to imagine your new self, to step into the future and see your future self, is a valuable tool on this healing journey.

The question is: can you see her? Can you feel her energy, even if just for a moment?

For the longest time, I couldn't. My vibration was so entrenched in victimhood that imagining myself as anything else felt like a fantasy, like playacting at being someone I could never actually become. But the truth is, that divine future self isn't something you become—it's something you remember. It's the frequency you were born with, the vibration you've temporarily forgotten.

Connecting with your divine future self becomes a powerful anchor point for raising your vibration. When you can see her, feel her, imagine stepping into her energy—even for just a few moments—you create a vibrational pathway between where you are now and where you're headed. You give your energy permission to shift in that direction. You change your vibrational compass direction.

This doesn't happen all at once. Keep in mind the compass analogy—just one degree of adjustment changes your entire trajectory. Each time you choose to see yourself through the eyes of your future divine self rather than through the lens of your victim story, you shift your vibration. Each time you catch yourself speaking from that victim frequency and consciously choose different words, different thoughts, different energy—you move up the ladder.

Step by step, you move toward the frequency of your divine self. And with each step, the vibration of victimhood loses its grip on you. You are rising up from the vibration of domestic violence—it no longer defines you; you are rising above it.

Part one tools & practices

The journey from victim to victor begins with the gentlest of steps. These foundational practices are designed to help you reconnect with the divine spark that has always existed within you, even when it felt buried beneath pain and trauma.

Start slowly. Be patient with yourself. Your nervous system has been in survival mode, and healing requires the tender care you would give a wounded bird learning to fly again.

Simple breathing technique - calm the nervous system

Whilst the body has been in fight, flight or freeze for so long, the breath has become shallow and quick. I remember feeling frustrated when someone told me to "just breathe". In the moment, it felt impossible. When we are stressed or traumatized, our breath becomes shallow and rapid, which keeps our nervous system on alert and in survival mode. Slow, deep breathing does the opposite—it signals to our brain that we're safe, activating our body's natural calming response. Here is a simple exercise that will help your body and your nervous system in these early days. I discuss more about the breath in *Part Three - I am Vibrant*.

1. Breathe in - take a deep breath through the nose into the very bottom of your belly and allow the belly to fill (push out) as you breathe in. If you feel like you can't do this, remind your body that it knows how to do this and just continue. Your body can and will remember how to allow a deep breath. Allow the breath to fill the belly and up to the chest to the count of about 5 seconds, pause and take one more "sip" of air*. You can watch a second hand on a clock or use a timer or metronome to time the seconds.
2. Breathe out – through the mouth, gently as though loosely blowing out a candle. Allow the belly to empty from the bottom as you breathe out and allow it to become deflated, pressing gently towards your backbone. Breathe out to the count of 7-8 seconds. Pause a moment before taking your next breath.

Repeat 3 times. You may notice a yawn or a calm affect in your body after you have done this.

* Use the "Sip" of air to calm when you are in a heightened state. For all other times, simply use the 3 deep breaths, five seconds in, eight seconds out.

Repeat this exercise as many times during the day as you need and for as many days in a row as you can. Each time it will remind your body that you are safe.

Release being a victim EFT tapping

This may be a difficult meditation to do. It may feel raw and emotional. There will likely be tears. That's all okay.

I remember this being difficult—it brought up so much more than I expected. When more comes up, acknowledge it. Write it down. Do a tapping on it later. For me, words like "failure", "idiot", "so stupid" all surfaced. All of these were rooted in victim mentality. I could have changed the word "victim" in the tapping to "failure" or anything else I felt at the time, but the victim tapping was still the most effective release of pent-up emotions, self-sabotaging habits, and limiting beliefs. I simply had to let go of the role of victim before I could move forward. In hindsight, I wish I had discovered this years earlier than I did.

Before you begin; refer to the EFT tapping information on *Page 165* of this book for explanations of the tapping points and more information about how the Emotional Freedom Technique works. Try the detailed tapping example for *Releasing Shame and Guilt*.

Find a quiet place where you will be undisturbed for about 15 minutes.

Take a deep belly breath and feel into what being a victim feels like. Say out loud "I am a victim".

Rate how true it feels on a scale of 1 – 10, 1 being I'm hardly a victim at all and 10 being in total victim mode. Allow that number to be there whatever it is with no judgement. It's ok.

You can tell yourself "It's ok that I am where I am right now, it's ok that I'm here".

Karate Chop - repeat 3 times while tapping - choose one, rotate all three, or choose your own specific statement.

"Even though I was a victim of abuse, I choose to reclaim my power now".

"Even though I've been living in victim identity, I'm ready to transform".

"Even though being the victim felt safe, I'm ready to step into my strength".

Round 1: Acknowledging
EB - I am such a victim
SE - That part is real and undeniable
UE - I lived through something terrible
UN - I was hurt and harmed
CH - This victim identity kept me safe
CB – But it's become a prison of its own
UA - I should never have had to go through this pain
CR – I'm afraid no one will believe it happened if I'm not a victim anymore

Take a deep breath and release.

Round 2: Leaning Toward Letting Go
KC – Even though I am a victim, I am open to releasing being a victim now
EB - What if I could honour what happened without staying stuck?
SE - I can acknowledge I was victimized without being a victim

UE - That was something that happened to me, not who I am
UN - I'm ready to release this identity
CH - I'm more than what was done to me
CB - I survived, and that makes me a survivor not a victim
UA - I can be strong and still honour my pain
CR - Letting go of the victim story
Take a deep breath and release.

Round 3: Empowerment
KC – What if I honour what happened and choose to move forward?
EB - I am not a victim, I am a survivor
SE - I choose to reclaim my power
UE - I define myself now, not my past
UN - I am strong, capable, and whole
CH - My story is one of resilience, not defeat
CB - I am the author of my life now
UA - I choose empowerment over victimhood
CR - I reclaim my strength
Take a deep breath and release. Notice how you feel now.

Say out loud, "I am a victim". Rate – 0-10. Repeat the tapping if you are still above a 2-3.

Repeat this tapping meditation in the coming week. You might like to leave it a day or two before repeating the exercise. After you have done it 3 – 4 times, notice where you feel a difference in your body. Journal any success, notice how other people interact with you.

Awareness practice

This is a simple and powerful exercise that I use throughout my life still. Simply say to yourself as many times a day as you remember, "I am aware". Write it on a sticky note on your bathroom mirror, by the tea kettle or in your office space. This powerful phrase will help increase your awareness and becoming aware opens you to infinite possibilities. You will notice yourself becoming more aware of your feelings, other people's energies, the energies around you. You will become more aware of the divine nature that is you and become aware of small shifts in your life. You will become aware of when you are tensing, when you feel "heavy" or when you are feeling "lighter" and more at ease. Becoming aware allows you to choose in any moment the frequency you want to focus your attention on.

PART TWO – I AM INTELLIGENT

Trusting our intuition and rebuilding confidence in our decisions.

Domestic violence creates a profound disruption to our natural intelligence—our innate ability to collect, process, and effectively use information. One of the phrases I have remembered through most of my life is this: "high emotion, low intelligence". Fundamentally, the human brain cannot operate both hemispheres at full capacity simultaneously. The emotional centres and the rational thinking centres compete for resources. Although both can work together in harmony, when emotions run high, our access to rational thought becomes limited. When we exist in a state of chronic stress and hypervigilance, our cognitive resources become hijacked by survival mechanisms. The constant threat assessment required in an abusive environment fragments our attention, making it difficult to think clearly, make sound decisions, or access our full intellectual capacity.

Our brains, designed to protect us, shift into reactive patterns that prioritize immediate safety over analytical thinking. This survival mode, while necessary for protection, can leave us feeling scattered, forgetful, and disconnected from our inner wisdom. The trauma of abuse creates neural pathways focused on threat detection rather than creative problem-solving or strategic planning. Recognizing this impact is the first step toward reclaiming our mental clarity and rebuilding trust in our own intelligence.

Compounding this disruption is the insidious tactic of gaslighting—a deliberate manipulation where the perpetrator systematically denies our reality, twists our words, and questions our perception of events until we begin to doubt not only our own intelligence, but our sanity. When someone repeatedly tells us that what we experienced didn't happen, that we're "too sensitive", "overreacting", "or "remembering it wrong", our natural intelligence becomes further fragmented. We lose trust not just in our memories, but in our ability to perceive reality accurately. This erosion of self-trust is intentional—it keeps us confused, dependent, and unable to think clearly enough to recognize the abuse for what it is or to plan our escape. Gaslighting doesn't just damage our confidence; it actively dismantles our cognitive ability to function, leaving us questioning every thought, feeling, and decision we make.

Transforming the Root System

As we begin to understand how domestic violence fragments our natural intelligence, we must also recognize that true healing requires us to examine and transform the deep-rooted beliefs stored in our subconscious mind—those powerful roots that have been nourishing thoughts of brokenness, inadequacy, and victimhood. Like a magnificent tree, our conscious efforts to rebuild our lives represent only the visible growth; the real transformation happens when we tend to the root system of our beliefs.

Understanding our own patterns is crucial to breaking free and ensuring abuse never happens again. As we release these limiting beliefs and victim stories, our energy shifts to an entirely new frequency. Our reclaimed intelligence—no longer hijacked by survival mode—can now operate from a place of clarity, wisdom, and empowered choice. This is how we ensure that what happened before will never happen again: not through vigilance or fear, but through the complete transformation of our energetic signature.

The Power of the Subconscious Mind

Beneath the surface of our conscious awareness lies the subconscious, a vast and intricate network of beliefs, perceptions, and experiences that silently orchestrate the majority of our daily existence. Like a magnificent tree, what we observe of our mental processes—the visible trunk, branches, and leaves of our conscious thoughts—represents only a fraction of what truly governs our inner world. The subconscious mind is that vast network of roots spreading deep beneath the surface, holding the real power in nourishing and shaping how we navigate through life.

Research suggests that the subconscious mind governs approximately 90-95% of our daily life, leaving only 5% under our conscious control. This means that the vast majority of our decisions, actions, emotions, and behaviours operate on autopilot, driven by deeply embedded programs and beliefs that run below our awareness. Like a plane flying on autopilot, our subconscious manages everything from how we walk and breathe to how we think and what we believe about ourselves. This serves us well—we don't need to wake each day and relearn how to talk or walk, tie a shoe, or make a sandwich. These programs have been worn in like a well-used bush track. But this autopilot can work against us when the subconscious has programmed beliefs and patterns that no longer serve us—or worse, actively harm us. This is why conscious effort alone isn't enough to create lasting transformation after domestic violence; real change requires addressing the subconscious programming that controls most of our experience.

Understanding Subconscious Patterns

These subconscious patterns were primarily formed during childhood—between birth and age seven—when our brains operated predominantly in theta brainwave states, essentially recording everything without the filter of critical thinking. Every repeated experience, emotional reaction, parental comment, and observed behaviour became encoded as neural pathways that now trigger automatically in similar situations.

These subconscious beliefs act as invisible architects of our reality, shaping everything from our self-worth and relationship dynamics to our financial ceiling and health outcomes. The challenge is that many of these programs are limiting or even contradictory to our conscious desires—we might consciously want success while subconsciously believing we're unworthy, or desire intimacy while unconsciously expecting abandonment. Becoming aware of these hidden patterns requires detective work: noticing recurring life themes, emotional triggers, self-sabotaging behaviours, and the gap between what we say we want and what we actually create.

Changing the Subconscious Program

The truth is, we are Divine. We are Intelligent. We are Vibrant. We are Authentic. We are already all of this, but we just don't believe it. When we don't believe it, we cannot live it. How do we shape this new belief and change the old beliefs of "not worthy" and "not good enough" and "not ___" and "not ___" and "not ___"? We need to tap into the subconscious and change the program.

Reprogramming the subconscious requires speaking its native language—not logic and willpower, but repetition, emotion, and altered states of consciousness. The most powerful access points occur during theta brainwave states: the drowsy moments just before sleep and upon waking, meditation, and states of emotion or presence. Techniques like visualization with emotional engagement, affirmations repeated with feeling rather than rote memorization, and embodiment practices that create new somatic experiences can bypass the critical conscious mind and write new programs directly into the subconscious. The key is consistency and emotional authenticity; the subconscious responds not to what we think we should believe, but to what we repeatedly feel and embody as true.

For those of us healing from domestic violence, the trauma often lives not just in our minds but in our bodies—locked into our nervous system, our muscles, our very cells. This is where techniques like EFT tapping become invaluable, helping to release trauma stored in the body that keeps old patterns locked in place, allowing the subconscious to finally let go of what it's been holding onto for our protection.

The subconscious can also be engaged in direct conversation through intentional inner dialogue, a practice that transforms the relationship from adversarial to collaborative. By entering a relaxed, meditative state and addressing the subconscious with respect—as we would a protective inner guardian rather than an enemy—we can ask it revealing questions: "What are you trying to protect me from by holding onto this belief?" or "What do you need from me to feel safe enough to release this pattern?". I often ask my subconscious if it can "see" the problem or pattern and I nearly always get a "yes" response.

This approach acknowledges that every subconscious program, no matter how limiting, was created with positive intent—usually protection, love, or survival. When we can thank these old programs for their service and explain that circumstances have changed, the subconscious often becomes willing to let them go. We might write letters to our subconscious, use automatic writing where we ask questions with our dominant hand and let our subconscious answer with our non-dominant hand, or simply speak aloud during those theta-state moments, giving permission to release what no longer serves us. The subconscious responds particularly well to gratitude, reassurance, and being given a new, upgraded belief to install in place of the old one. The subconscious doesn't like to be left empty, so giving it a new belief is important so it knows it can still keep us safe.

How My Beliefs Were Formed

The events and circumstances that moulded my understanding of the world came from countless sources: society's expectations, my immediate environment, family dynamics, cultural norms, educational experiences (like that teacher telling me I must be stupid), and the subtle messages absorbed from media and peers. Each interaction, each moment of triumph or disappointment, each whispered comment or raised eyebrow became a building block in the construction of my internal belief system and ultimately the building of my subconscious.

Over the years, I had accumulated what I came to think of as a "caddy of beliefs and perceptions"—a collection of mental tools and assumptions that my subconscious mind would automatically reach for whenever I encountered a situation requiring interpretation or response. I was out of touch with my divine self and allowed the subconscious to run on auto. This caddy contained everything from deeply held convictions about my own worth and capabilities to subtle biases about how the world operates and what I could expect from other people.

The remarkable thing about this subconscious repository is how efficiently it operates. Without any conscious effort on my part, it would instantly categorize new experiences, predict outcomes, and trigger emotional responses based on patterns it had learned from my past. A facial expression from a colleague might instantly activate memories of childhood criticism, causing me to feel defensive before I even understood why. A particular scent could transport me back to a moment of safety and comfort, influencing my mood and decisions in ways I couldn't immediately recognize.

This subconscious programming doesn't merely influence our reactions—it actively shapes our reality. It determines what we notice and what we overlook, what opportunities we perceive, and which ones remain invisible to us.

The beliefs stored in this mental caddy had become the lens through which I viewed everything. They determined whether I saw challenges as opportunities for growth or threats to be avoided, whether I approached relationships with openness or guardedness, whether I felt deserving of success or unconsciously sabotaged my own efforts. They ran the show so completely that I often felt like I was watching my own life happen to me, wondering why I kept ending up in uncomfortable situations or why certain patterns seemed to repeat themselves regardless of my conscious intentions.

Understanding this hidden architecture of the mind was both humbling and liberating. It explained why willpower alone so often failed to create lasting change, and why the most profound transformations seemed to happen not through force of conscious effort, but through somehow accessing and reshaping these deeper layers of belief and perception. This is where I had tried repeatedly and failed so many times to make lasting change in my life. It wasn't until I began to study the subconscious mind—and in particular my belief systems—that I was able to make changes that truly stuck.

My subconscious mind, I realized, was not my enemy but rather my devoted guardian that had been doing its best to protect and guide me based on the information it had gathered throughout my life. The challenge was learning to communicate with this part of myself, to update its outdated programming, and to consciously participate in the ongoing formation of the beliefs that would continue to shape my reality.

The Power of Language and Belief

Our subconscious beliefs don't just operate in isolation. They actively shape how we perceive and interpret every experience, and most importantly, they influence the very words we choose to describe our reality. These deeply embedded programs act like invisible filters, determining not only what we notice in any given moment, but how we make meaning from it and express it through language.

When our subconscious holds beliefs rooted in victimhood or powerlessness, we unconsciously select words that reinforce these limiting patterns, speaking about ourselves and our experiences—including those who have harmed us—in ways that keep us energetically bound to lower frequencies. But here's where our power lies: by becoming conscious of this connection between belief, perception, and language, we can begin to deliberately choose words that reflect our highest truth rather than our wounded past.

This is where we move from unconscious reaction to conscious creation, from victim to DIVA. The question becomes not just "What do I believe?" but "How am I speaking my beliefs into existence, and are these words lifting me up or holding me back?". When we understand that our language is both a reflection of our inner world and a creative force shaping our outer reality, we can begin to wield it as the powerful tool of transformation it truly is.

The Power of Shifting Perspective

One of the most profound shifts in reclaiming my "already there" intelligence came through learning to question my initial reactions and perspectives. I discovered two simple but powerful questions that completely transformed how I processed difficult experiences: "Is this true?" and "How can I see this differently?".

These questions became my gateway to breaking free from the automatic, fear-based interpretations my subconscious mind had been running on autopilot for years. When something triggered me—whether it was a memory from my past, a challenging interaction with someone, or even my own harsh self-judgment—instead of accepting my first emotional reaction as absolute truth, I learned to pause and ask these questions.

The first question, "Is this true?" created space between me and my immediate reaction. It allowed me to step back and examine whether the story my mind was telling me in the present moment was actually factual or simply a familiar pattern based on old programming. As Seneca wisely noted, "We suffer more in imagination than in reality," and I was beginning to see how much additional suffering I was creating through my interpretations of current situations—separate from the very real trauma I had experienced.

Often, I discovered, that what felt absolutely true in the moment was actually an interpretation filtered through my past experiences and limiting beliefs. An example of testing this for ourselves can simply be a matter of checking in after a thought that comes across as a statement, like, "this always happens to me". Is this true? Does this really always happen?

The second question, "How can I see this differently?" opened up entirely new perspectives and possibilities. This wasn't about forcing myself to think positively or denying legitimate concerns—it was about expanding my perspective beyond the narrow, fear-based view that trauma had conditioned me to default to. Sometimes this shift in perspective revealed opportunities I couldn't see before, helped me understand another person's actions with more compassion, or simply freed me from the emotional prison of my initial interpretation.

These simple questions became tools of liberation, allowing me to access the intelligent, clear-thinking part of myself that had been overshadowed by reactive patterns. Each time I used them, I strengthened my ability to respond from wisdom rather than react from wounds.

Choosing Words That Elevate

The language we use to describe our experiences carries tremendous energetic weight, particularly when discussing those who have harmed us. While it may feel natural to use harsh or vengeful words about a perpetrator, doing so keeps us energetically bound to lower frequencies of anger and resentment. When we speak with hatred or contempt, we're not just describing external reality—we're creating an internal vibration that affects our entire being.

Try this awareness exercise now: speak a negative, harsh word aloud and notice how it feels in our body—the tension, the constriction, the heaviness. Now speak a word of compassion, strength, or hope, and observe the different sensation—perhaps expansion, lightness, or warmth. This isn't about excusing harmful behaviour or bypassing legitimate anger; it's about recognizing that we have the power to choose words that elevate rather than diminish our energy. When we consciously select language that reflects our highest self, we step into our power as creators of our own energetic environment, moving from victim consciousness toward the sovereignty of a true DIVA.

The Language of Self-Talk

The language we use to speak to ourselves and to our body carries immense power. While we may feel justified in "kicking ourselves" for getting into a difficult situation—"How could I be so stupid?!"—this harsh internal dialogue doesn't help our cells heal or our mind recover. The words we choose in our self-talk become the foundation of our healing journey, and understanding this connection is crucial for moving from victim to victor.

Remember this; it was not our fault that this happened. It was not our fault at all. The sooner we can ease up on ourselves and step away from the blame game, the sooner real healing can begin.

That said, we can also acknowledge that our choices and actions, influenced by our subconscious programming and limiting beliefs, led us into that situation. This isn't about blame—the abuse was never our responsibility. But recognizing that we made certain choices from a place of unworthiness or unhealed wounds is actually empowering. It means we have the power to make different choices now. Understanding this distinction allows us to take ownership of our future without carrying shame about our past.

Perpetrators of domestic violence are skilled manipulators who carefully select their victims—not only for weaknesses, but for specific vulnerabilities. They look for qualities like empathy, loyalty, the desire to help others, or perhaps someone going through a transitional period in life. These aren't character flaws; they're often some of our most beautiful human qualities, twisted and exploited by someone with harmful intentions.

Yes, we made choices that led us into that situation. We all make choices based on the information we have at the time, our past experiences, and our emotional state. But the way we were treated—the abuse, the manipulation, the cruelty—is not a reflection of our intelligence or our worth as people. It's a reflection of the perpetrator's character, not ours.

During my own healing journey, I discovered how the harsh words I used against myself gradually transformed into deeply held beliefs. I believed it was my fault somehow. I carried shame for "allowing" myself to be treated in such a way. I felt overwhelming guilt that I didn't "get out" earlier. I felt very stupid.

These weren't just passing thoughts—they became the lens through which I viewed myself and my experience. The language of self-criticism created a secondary layer of trauma, one that I was inflicting on myself long after I had escaped the physical situation.

Our brains don't distinguish between the harsh criticism we receive from others and the harsh criticism we give ourselves. When we repeatedly tell ourselves we're stupid, weak, or at fault, our nervous system responds as if we're under attack. This keeps us in a state of hypervigilance and stress, making healing exponentially more difficult.

Conversely, when we speak to ourselves with compassion and accuracy about what happened, we create space for genuine healing. This isn't about positive thinking or pretending everything is fine—it's about replacing untruths with truth, shame with understanding, and self-attack with self-compassion.

Intelligence Beyond the Mind

While we often think of intelligence as something that happens only in our heads, our bodies possess their own sophisticated intelligence systems. From the neural networks in our hearts to the gut's "second brain", our entire being is designed to process information, make decisions, and guide us toward healing. Understanding this broader definition of intelligence helps us tap into the wisdom that exists throughout our entire system—not just in our thinking minds.

Our emotions can be used as a guidance system, alerting us to moments when we are in fight or flight and allowing us to relax into accessing our divine intelligence, no matter what we are facing. Remember the phrase "high emotion, low intelligence", meaning when we are in a highly emotional state, we do not have access to our divine intelligence. One of our uniquely human abilities is to step out of the "high emotion, low intelligence" cycle and into "high intelligence, low emotion"—becoming conscious observers of our own existence and perceptions. But understanding this isn't enough—we must learn to apply it.

True intelligence, at its very core, is about gathering knowledge and then applying it meaningfully. When we use our intelligence to understand how our body systems actually work and the intricate dance between our body's systems, emotions and our stress responses, we can then apply this understanding to transform our lived experience. In addition, accessing divine intelligence adds yet a deeper level from which we can operate. From this place of informed clarity, we move beyond simply reacting to life and begin consciously creating the lives we truly want.

This realization became my lifeline during one of the most challenging aspects of my recovery. When we are acquiring knowledge and then using it, we are using our intelligence—we are therefore intelligent. This simple truth became my anchor when I went through the hardest time with the belief that I was either no longer intelligent or never had intelligence due to the decisions I had made. How could I be smart if I had gotten myself into a situation where I was living with domestic violence? The struggles I incurred after that experience further cemented the belief that I lacked intelligence. I no longer trusted myself, my decisions, or my choices.

But by then, I had so many other tools behind me that this became something I could work on. Using the powerful questions—"Is this true?" and "How can I see this differently?"—I began to challenge this belief about my intelligence. I questioned everything: Is this belief mine or someone else's? Is this going to work for me? How does this idea feel in my body? Through this process, I began to uncover the meaning of the words I was using and the affirmations I had created.

The interesting work of Dr. Masaru Emoto had inspired me to delve deeper into the language I was using. If the word "peace" spoken to water created microscopic structures of beauty, while other lower vibrational words created no such structures, then what were all the words I was using doing to my body and my world? If I could say the words "love" and "idiot" to jars of rice in water and see physical changes, what was happening in my own mind and body? I became curious.

Having curiosity about everything is a large part of our intelligence, and being open to exploring more for our own development is vital. I encourage anyone reading this book to seek to study more about the topics and ideas in addition to using the practices. However, I did need to learn the balance between curiosity and wanting to learn more to "fix" all the broken parts of me. I found that when I had a physical ailment, I immediately delved so deep into it that I would end up in some kind of rabbit hole. Suddenly my energy was off, I was desperate and trying too hard again.

Opening to Infinite Possibilities

Sometimes we have a thought about how we want things to work out, how we want things to go, but often these thoughts are coming from a very limited, restricted perspective—and often from a place where we are subconsciously and desperately trying to keep safe. When we are in crisis, all we can see is the worst and all we can do is hope for not the worst. But there is more available than just hope. The goal here is to allow something better. To soften into it and surrender to allowing something better than what we could have ever hoped for or imagined.

Ask ourselves: "What's the best that can happen?". As we stop trying to force an outcome that we think is going to feel good, that we think is going to be for our best, then the best becomes possible. I have practiced this several times with amazing outcomes—far better outcomes than what I thought possible from my very limited view at the time.

In a very desperate situation, highly emotional and frightening, I became aware of myself tensing up in my body. My breath could hardly squeeze in and out of my lungs, my throat and chest felt tight. Terror caused my body to freeze, and I waited. Then I had one single thought that felt wrong in that moment: "What is the best that can happen for me right now?".

The rest of my mind was screaming at me, "What the hell, lady—we are about to die and there is no best!". There were times when, yes, I was in danger and I believed I would die, but in other moments it was totally my mind running from something that was not going to kill me in that moment. When that foreign little thought, "what's the best that can happen?" crept in from somewhere and just settled itself like a cat curling up on my lap, I felt a calmness within my body.

I began to relax by about 1%, but as we know, the smallest shift can be groundbreaking. I was able to breathe in, and as I focused on that question in my mind, it grew slightly more powerful: "What is the best that can happen for me right now?". And so, I was able to, in a moment of despair and fear, shift the energy. I was able to shift my vibration. That energy shift, that moment of allowing, brought a change so powerful that to this day, I am still in awe about it. The situation changed suddenly and in a way I never thought possible.

Possibilities in the universe are endless. Endless possibilities, infinite possibilities. With our human mind designed for survival, we are very often unable to reach those possibilities in moments of despair because we have created a kink, if you like, in the flow of allowing. Our powerful minds, focusing on just one small aspect and creating more of what we don't want, creates a kink in the energy—like a garden hose that gets twisted and blocks the water flow.

When we open up the flow of allowing and are open to a different possibility, one can easily become available to us. In addition to "What is the best that can happen?" asking "What's possible here?" is even more expansive because we are then accessing something far greater than the situation we are looking at.

But when we are in a moment of physical danger, our number one priority is to stay safe. That's more than perfectly okay. But also allow that possibility, allow that question to linger. Ask ourselves: "what is the solution?". When we ask that question, we shift our energy from being deep in a problem and move into being in the energy of the solution. These options all sound ridiculously simple, but the power of the intention of finding out is immense.

I recall one incident of such violence; I was afraid to open my eyes. This almost daily feeling of fear had become my norm. I was exhausted. At the time, I closed my eyes and sobbed, defeated, waiting for whatever blow was coming. I was frozen. And in my mind, I was saying over and over, "I am safe, I am okay." I didn't know what else to do. I never fought back, knowing if I tried it would be worse the next time, so I made myself small to minimize the impact and kept repeating "I am safe, I am okay."

It was a lie. I was not safe and I knew it, and every repetition of this tiny affirmation seemed to cement the fact that I was not safe. In that moment, other options were completely unavailable to me. I was completely in the problem, unable to get into the space of the solution, having no knowledge of possibilities or the best that could happen.

When I reflect back on these two different thought patterns in similar situations—asking "what's the best that can happen?" versus desperately repeating "I am safe"—the power of my thoughts was clear. In the first situation, that single question shifted my energy enough that the entire situation dissolved in a way I never thought possible. In the second, the affirmation that contradicted my reality kept me locked in fear, frozen and waiting for the next blow. The difference wasn't in the words themselves, but in whether those words opened a doorway to possibility or slammed against the wall of my current truth.

But these experiences also taught me something crucial about affirmations. They aren't wrong—they're simply tools, and like any tool, they work better in some situations than others. When we use affirmations that don't feel true, our inner wisdom knows the difference. If saying "I am safe" when we're clearly not safe creates internal resistance, that's our truth trying to protect us. And so that kink seems tighter.

The key is to bridge the gap between where we are and where we want to be. Instead of forcing an affirmation that feels like a lie, try these gentler approaches:

"What if I could be safe?", "I want to feel safe", "I am open to finding safety", "I am learning to recognize safety", "I am worthy of safety".

These statements don't ask us to deny our current reality—they create space for possibility without demanding that we believe something that contradicts our experience.

Traditional affirmations work beautifully when there's alignment between what we're saying and what feels possible. But when there's a big gap, softer language creates a bridge instead of a wall. The goal isn't to convince ourselves of something untrue—it's to open our mind to what could become true.

The idea here is to keep asking these possibility-focused questions in as many situations as possible, so they become our go-to responses. They become available instantly, like a well-worn path in our mind that leads toward hope rather than deeper into despair.

Future Memory: Rewiring Our Internal Timeline

For so long, my memories held me hostage. Every trigger pulled me backward into scenes I desperately wanted to forget—the arguments, the fear, the moments I felt powerless. My brain had become a museum of trauma, replaying the past on an endless loop. But then I discovered something revolutionary: if I could vividly remember the past, I could just as vividly remember my future.

Where focus goes, energy flows. This isn't just a platitude—it's a fundamental truth about how our consciousness creates our reality. When we continuously focus on the past, replaying our trauma stories and reliving those painful moments, we place ourselves in vibrational alignment with more of the same. Our energy, our attention, our very life force gets poured into what has already happened, and the universe responds by bringing us more experiences that match that frequency. The more we loop through the old stories, the more we strengthen the neural pathways that keep us trapped in victim consciousness, magnetizing situations and relationships that mirror our internal state.

Future memory isn't about denying what happened or pretending the past doesn't exist—it's about consciously choosing where to place our attention and energy. Instead of constantly revisiting who I was in my darkest moments, I began meditating into my future self. I would close my eyes and step into her—the woman I was becoming. I could feel her confidence, her peace, her joy. I could see her surroundings, sense how she moved through her day, hear the way she spoke to herself with kindness.

The more I practiced remembering this future, the more my nervous system began to relax into it, recognizing it as familiar rather than foreign. My brain started treating these future memories with the same weight it had given my traumatic past, except these memories pulled me forward instead of dragging me back. This shift in focus became one of my most powerful healing tools—I was no longer defined by where I'd been but magnetized by where I was going.

Reclaiming our intelligence after domestic violence is not about becoming smarter or just learning new information—it's about remembering what was always there. Our intelligence was never broken; it was hijacked by survival mechanisms that kept us alive. As we clear the fog of trauma, reprogram our subconscious beliefs, choose language that elevates rather than diminishes, and shift our focus from past wounds to future possibilities, we don't create intelligence—we reveal it. We step back into our natural state of clarity, wisdom, and divine knowing. This is the intelligence of a DIVA: not intellectual prowess measured by external standards, but the profound wisdom that comes from knowing ourselves completely, trusting our inner guidance, and consciously creating our reality from a place of empowered choice. Our intelligence was never the question. Our willingness to reclaim it, trust it, and use it to build the life we deserve—that is where our true power lies

Part two tools & practices

Intelligence is in a nutshell, the acquisition and use of knowledge. Knowledge without application remains merely information. The following practices and exercises are designed to help you move beyond understanding these concepts intellectually and begin embodying them in your daily life. Through heart-centred meditation, you'll learn to access your divine intelligence, that innate wisdom that exists beyond the trauma and conditioning. You'll explore how your beliefs shape your reality. Most importantly, you'll harness the transformative power of language itself, learning how the words you speak and think can literally rewire your neural pathways and create new possibilities. These aren't just theoretical concepts—they're practical tools for reclaiming your power and stepping fully into your role as the intelligent and conscious creator of your life.

Three way alignment meditation

This meditation brings your three intelligence centres—your brain, heart, and gut—into rhythmic alignment.

When these centres synchronize through slow, intentional focus on the heart and breath, you shift from stress and scattered thinking into an aligned state of calm, clarity, and deeper intuition.

(For more information about the heart, brain, gut connection and the science behind this practice, go to the Additional Information section.)

1. Slow the breath. Breathe in through the nose for 5 seconds and out through the mouth for 7-8 seconds. This reminds the body it is safe. Do this for a minute or two, keeping your rhythm slow and consistent.
2. Place a flat hand on your belly, just below the navel.
3. Place your other hand over the centre of your chest. Feel your heartbeat. I like to use my fingertips on my sternum. Place your attention on your heart, the feeling of it beating and at the same time focus on breathing slowly and deeply.
4. As you breathe in, imagine the breath is love, light and appreciation flowing into your heart. You can say the words "love" or "thank you".
5. As you breathe out, imagine you are breathing love, light and appreciation out of your heart and into every cell in your body.
6. Stay in this meditation for 5-10 minutes, whatever feels comfortable, ensuring your attention is on your heart while focusing on the breath. If your attention wanders, gently bring it back.

7. You can stop here if you like or while in this state you can ask a question. You have access to your divine intelligence and intuition from this space. Some answers may come later, some immediately. Either way is fine but ensure you don't try too hard. Soften into the process, trust it and allow.

Identifying and changing Beliefs exercise

A belief is a thought we feel in our body to be true. And some of the beliefs we carry—the ones we absorbed from family, society, past trauma—are lies that our bodies have learned to accept as fact. When we live through these beliefs, our life is limited. Example,

Belief: money is hard to come by.

Limit: not enough money.

This exercise will help you identify those limiting beliefs, understand where they came from, and begin the process of releasing them.

What You'll Need:

- A quiet space where you won't be interrupted
- Paper and pen
- 20-30 minutes

Before you start take three deep, aware belly breaths, in for the count of 5, out for the count of 8. Allow the belly to expand on the in breath and deflate on the out breath.

Step 1: Identify a limiting belief - Ask, "what limiting beliefs are active in my body right now?" or try these prompts.

"I am not enough because..."
"I can't have/do/be because..."
"Other people see me as not enough because..."

Don't filter or judge what comes up. Write quickly. Let the beliefs flow onto the page, even if they seem silly or contradictory. Examples might include:

- "I am not enough because I'm not married"
- "I am not enough because I don't earn six figures"
- "I am not enough because I'm not thin enough"

Step 2: Find the Root - Look at your list. Circle the beliefs that feel the most charged—the ones that make your chest tighten or your stomach drop. Pick your top three.

For each one, ask: *"Where did I learn this? Who taught me this was true?"*

Write down the memories, people, or moments that come to mind.

Step 3: Challenge the Belief - For each circled belief, answer these questions:

- Is this true for me?
- What evidence do I have that contradicts this belief?
- Would I say this to my best friend if she believed it about herself?
- Who benefits from me believing this about myself?

Step 4: Rewrite the Truth - For each limiting belief, write a new truth. Make it present tense, personal, and powerful.

Old belief: "I am not enough because I'm not married"
New truth: "I am whole and complete exactly as I am. My worth exists independent of any relationship".

Step 5: Release This part is physical and symbolic. Choose one:

- Tear up the page with your old beliefs and throw it away (or burn it safely)
- Cross out each limiting belief with a thick black marker
- Write your new truths on a fresh page and place it somewhere you'll see daily
- Or simply say out loud, "I now release this old belief"

Moving Forward: These beliefs didn't form overnight, and they won't disappear overnight either. When an old belief surfaces (and it will), acknowledge it: "There's that old story again". Then consciously choose your new truth instead. With practice, your body will begin to feel the new truth just as deeply as it once felt the old lie.

Future memory exercise - meet your future self.

Instead of dwelling on the past, what if you could remember your future? What if the woman you're becoming is already waiting for you, and all you need to do is meet her?

This exercise will help you connect with the strongest, most empowered version of yourself—not as a distant dream, but as a memory you're stepping into.

What You'll Need:

- 15-20 minutes of quiet time
- A comfortable place to sit or lie down
- Paper and pen for afterward

The Exercise:

Close your eyes and take three deep breaths. Let your body settle.

Now, imagine yourself five years from now. You've done the work. You've healed. You've become the woman you were always meant to be.

See her clearly:

- Where is she? What does her home look like?
- How does she carry herself? How does she move through the world?
- What does her daily life look like?
- Who is around her? What relationships has she cultivated?
- What does she no longer tolerate?
- What brings her joy?

Notice how she feels in her body—confident, grounded, free. This isn't fantasy. This is memory. You're remembering who you become.

Now, let her speak to you. What does your future self want you to know? What advice does she have? What does she want to thank you for doing today?

Listen. Really listen.

When you're ready, open your eyes and write down everything you remember about her—the details, the feelings, her message to you.

Living Your Future Memory:

Keep this description somewhere you can see it. This isn't a goal to chase—it's a memory to step into. Every day, ask yourself: "What would my future self do right now?", then do that.

You're not becoming her. You're remembering her. And with each choice, each boundary, each act of self-love, you're proving that memory true.

PART THREE – I AM VIBRANT

Restoring our physical and mental health and embracing joyful living.

When I think of vibrance and being vibrant, I think of the sense that my mind, body, and spirit are working together harmoniously. That all my elements are at their best health, their highest vibration.

When you are vibrant physically, the fog that trauma created clears. It's thinking clearly without the fog of chronic stress clouding your mind. Your thoughts feel organized rather than scattered, and you can focus on what matters instead of constantly scanning for danger. Decision-making becomes easier when your nervous system isn't hijacked by survival mode.

Proper nutrition stabilizes blood sugar, which stabilizes mood. Movement releases endorphins and processes stress hormones. Quality sleep allows the brain to consolidate healing and form new, healthier neural pathways. Mental clarity emerges as the body finds balance. When you're no longer running on survival mode, your mind can focus on creation rather than protection. Decision-making becomes clearer. Self-trust grows stronger.

Emotional stability follows physical care. A regulated nervous system can hold bigger emotions without overwhelm. You begin to feel your feelings fully rather than fear them.

Spiritual connection deepens as you inhabit your body with love rather than fear. Your body becomes a sacred temple again—a place where your divine essence can fully express itself.

Vibrant health is waking up naturally refreshed, with energy that flows steadily throughout the day. It's having the physical stamina to engage fully with life, to play, to love, and to pursue those outrageous feel-good dreams. It's sharing with others, giving and receiving and being an active part of life itself.

Joy feels genuine and there is no guilt about feeling happy. Thoughts feel organized, decisions easy and intuition is alive. As you heal one aspect, you heal them all. Your vibrancy isn't something you lost—it's something you're remembering how to access.

My Journey Back to Feeling Good

Doesn't it feel good to feel good! A few years ago, this phrase had absolutely no meaning to me. I had forgotten what it felt like to feel good, and feeling good seemed so far removed from my reality that I had resigned myself to feeling less than average and to the chronic illnesses that had manifested in my body. I was also incredibly confused about my health. In my mind, I had escaped the domestic violence situation, so I should have been feeling amazing. I wasn't.

The biggest issue for me was a chronic skin condition that developed on my feet about six months after leaving. The condition worsened to the point where it was painful for me to walk. My skin was split and covered with blisters, ulcers, and open weeping sores on the soles of my feet and around my ankles. I tried every type of cream, soak, and wash I could find, but nothing worked.

Stepping onto the carpet each morning as I got out of bed felt like walking on hot coals or broken glass. Pain shot through my legs from the very first step of the day. Wearing closed shoes caused just as many problems as wearing sandals. It defeated me completely. I remember going to the doctor and asking if a skin graft was possible. At another visit years later, I had quite seriously through sobs, asked if amputation might be an option. I didn't want the pain anymore; I didn't want my feet anymore. I wanted out of this painful situation. I had endured enough pain in my life, and this felt like too much. With no known cure for this type of skin condition, I was told by doctors I would have to manage the symptoms as best I could for the rest of my life. I simply didn't have the energy to feel this much pain anymore. I was desperate.

In addition, I was having heart issues, breathing issues and digestive issues. I ended up in hospital more than once—I felt afraid I would die from whatever illness was plaguing me. My whole body felt like it really was broken, shutting down, tired, exhausted. And as life was going on seemingly without me, I did not have the time to lay down and sleep for days and weeks to allow time for healing and rest. I didn't even have time to be in hospital for an overnight.

I have always been a believer in "healthy mind, healthy body," so when my body wasn't functioning the way I wanted it to, when it wasn't healthy and I didn't feel good, I set out on a path to discover what I could do with my mind to change this. I was inspired by Dr Joe Dispenza's story of how he healed his broken spine, literally just with his thoughts. This journey into my personal health spanned many years. I studied extensively, and while this subject could easily be explored much deeper, for this discussion I'll break down my learnings and experience into smaller, digestible pieces.

Understanding what was happening in my body became the first step toward healing. I needed to know why my body was responding this way, and what I discovered changed everything.

How Domestic Violence Disrupts Your Nervous System

Domestic violence affects all aspects of health, and in my experience, these effects persist long after escaping the abusive situation. The impact of domestic violence on the body begins with the nervous system, which operates in two distinct modes.

The sympathetic nervous system is your body's alarm system, designed to keep you safe in moments of real danger. When it activates, your heart rate increases, breathing becomes shallow, muscles tense, and stress hormones flood your system. This "fight-or-flight" response is meant to be temporary, helping you escape danger or respond to an emergency. However, when you're living with domestic violence, this system stays switched on constantly, treating every moment as a potential threat.

The parasympathetic nervous system is your body's healing and restoration mode, often called "rest-and-digest." When this system is active, your heart rate slows, breathing deepens, muscles relax, and your body can focus on essential functions like digestion, immune response, and cellular repair. This is when true healing happens, both physically and emotionally. For survivors of domestic violence, learning to activate this system again is crucial for recovery, as the body needs to remember that it's safe to rest, heal, and simply be.

It's very easy to see that while the sympathetic nervous system is activated almost permanently and never switching off, the parasympathetic nervous system (needed to be active for the body to rejuvenate and repair) becomes dormant. The two do not function at the same time—it's one or the other.

The body and cells have memory, and learning to reactivate the parasympathetic nervous system is a process of reminding the body what its natural state of wellbeing is and how to find a way there.

The Amygdala: Your Brain's Alarm System

While the sympathetic and parasympathetic nervous systems orchestrate our body's overall response to stress and calm, there's a crucial brain structure that acts as the conductor of this physiological symphony. Deep within the limbic system lies the amygdala, a small but mighty almond-shaped cluster of neurons that serves as our brain's alarm system. This ancient structure doesn't just influence our nervous system responses—it essentially triggers them, determining in milliseconds whether we feel safe enough to rest and digest, or whether we need to prepare for action.

About the Amygdala: The amygdala processes emotional information with remarkable speed, often reacting to potential threats before our conscious mind even registers what's happening. It continuously scans our environment, evaluating sensory input against our stored memories of danger and safety. When it detects something potentially threatening—whether real or perceived—it instantly floods our system with stress hormones like adrenaline and cortisol, activating that sympathetic nervous system response.

Anxiety as Fear: Anxiety is fundamentally fear in disguise. While fear typically responds to immediate, identifiable threats, anxiety is fear's response to perceived future dangers or uncertainties. The amygdala doesn't distinguish between a genuine physical threat and an imagined worst-case scenario—it responds to both with the same intensity. This explains why someone can experience a full-blown panic response while simply thinking about or remembering a past trauma. The amygdala has essentially learned to fear the fear itself, creating cycles where anxiety about anxiety keeps the alarm system constantly activated.

For survivors of domestic violence, the amygdala often becomes hypervigilant, having learned that safety can disappear in an instant. Understanding this isn't weakness—it's your brain doing exactly what it was designed to do to keep you alive. However, this constant state of alert comes at a significant cost to your physical body. This is where understanding homeostasis becomes essential.

Understanding Homeostasis and Dis-ease

Homeostasis is the body's natural ability to maintain a stable, balanced internal environment despite changes happening around it. It is the body's built-in regulation system that keeps things like temperature, blood pressure, blood sugar, pH levels, and hormone levels within healthy ranges. When the body is in homeostasis, all your systems work harmoniously together—heart rate is steady, breathing is calm, the digestive system works properly, and the immune system functions optimally.

Domestic violence disrupts this natural state of health. It keeps the body locked in sympathetic nervous system dominance—fight-or-flight. When you're constantly in fight-or-flight mode, your body can't maintain homeostasis because it's too busy trying to survive perceived threats. The body goes into sympathetic nervous system mode and the chronic stress of being there throws all these delicate balancing systems out of whack. When these systems are out of balance, the body is susceptible to illness and dis-ease—the body's state of not being in a state of ease.

When the sympathetic nervous system is constantly activated, all body systems are affected. The immune system becomes compromised, and digestive function fails because the body cannot access the "rest and digest" mode of the parasympathetic nervous system. The immune system and digestive system are intimately connected—when one suffers, the other follows. Sleep becomes elusive when the body remains on high alert, again preventing access to the restorative parasympathetic state. From this condition of hypervigilance and chronic tension, with no opportunity for rest, muscle systems become strained and hormonal imbalances occur as stress hormones are overproduced. In a state of wellbeing, these stress hormones are only released at specific times and in small quantities.

Chronic inflammation develops throughout the body's systems, and illness takes hold. The cellular and body memory becomes reprogrammed to remain in survival mode, which meant for me that I continued living primarily through my sympathetic nervous system long after leaving the abusive environment. My body was indeed struggling, and I needed to begin to reactivate my parasympathetic system. As I started to understand what was happening in my body, I began to see how interconnected all these symptoms were. One of the most significant ways this hypervigilant state was showing up for me was in my digestive system, creating a vicious cycle that kept me trapped in dis-ease

The Gut-Brain Connection and Physical Symptoms

When your body perceives threat—whether real or remembered—it diverts energy away from non-essential functions like digestion to fuel your survival response. This creates a devastating cycle: chronic stress disrupts your digestive process, leading to poor nutrient absorption and cravings for quick energy fixes like sugar and processed foods. Your digestive system, which requires more energy to function properly than any other system in your body, becomes compromised and inefficient. I remember learning this in my ambulance officer training. I had gone out to an emergency with my team and our patient, involved in a serious car accident and badly injured, had thrown up. The body was stressed and the digestive system using the most energy, needed to be put on hold. Our bodies coming out of the DV environment can have constant issues with digestion as we still need to eat but the digestive system cannot function at full capacity while in stress mode.

Poor digestion then creates inflammation, nutrient deficiencies, and gut imbalances that affect every other system—your immune function, hormone production, and even your brain chemistry. When your body exists in this state of physical unwellness, it sends signals back to your mind that something is wrong, reinforcing that hypervigilant state and keeping you trapped in the very cycle that created the problem. The gut is named 'your second brain,' and when it's not functioning optimally, neither are you.

But the trap here is when the body isn't feeling well, we tend not to move it, and so begins another set of problems. Understanding the cost of staying still helped me see why movement became so essential to my healing.

The Hidden Cost of Staying Still

When we become sedentary, all kinds of symptoms can arise in the body. Without the proper flow of oxygen and blood, the digestive system slows, circulation slows, and our entire system begins to work less efficiently.

When our bodies remain still for extended periods, a cascade of changes begins to occur. Our cardiovascular system becomes less efficient, with the heart having to work harder to pump blood through vessels that have become less flexible. Muscle mass begins to decline—we can lose up to 3-5% of our muscle mass per decade after age 30 when inactive. Our bones become more brittle as they lose density without the stress that movement provides.

But perhaps most significantly for those of us recovering from trauma, lack of movement directly impacts our mental health. Physical inactivity disrupts the production of mood-regulating neurotransmitters like serotonin, dopamine, and endorphins—our body's natural "feel-good" chemicals. The stress hormone cortisol can remain elevated when we're sedentary, keeping us in a state of chronic tension. Research consistently shows that sedentary lifestyles are strongly linked to increased rates of depression and anxiety. Our bodies literally become stuck in patterns that mirror how we might feel emotionally trapped.

Once I understood what stillness was costing me, I was ready to discover what movement could give back.

The Magic of Movement

On the flip side, when we begin to move our bodies again, magic happens. Blood flow increases, delivering fresh oxygen and nutrients to every cell. Our lymphatic system—our body's cleanup crew—begins flowing more efficiently, helping to flush out toxins and waste. Muscles remember their strength and flexibility, joints begin to loosen, and we start to feel more at home in our own skin.

Movement triggers the release of endorphins—those wonderful natural mood elevators that can create feelings of euphoria and wellbeing. Regular movement also helps grow new brain cells and improves cognitive function. We literally think more clearly when we move regularly.

There's something profound that happens when we feel our muscles working, our heart pumping strong, our breath deepening. We remember that our body is not just a vessel for carrying pain—it's also a source of strength, pleasure, and vitality. We begin to trust our body again, to feel proud of what it can do rather than focusing on what it has endured.

Finding My Way Back Through Movement

Yes, some days it's difficult to get up and that's okay. Give yourself the time and space to just 'be' on those days, but other times, yes, you can absolutely give yourself a little nudge and get up and get moving. I found the best way to do this was to create a routine for myself that felt good for me. I went through so many illnesses and symptoms, and I began noticing I felt bad more often than I felt good. I started with some Qi Gong studies, because I not only wanted to get my body moving, I wanted to fix all the wrong bits. But as I studied, I realized I wasn't needing to fix anything that was wrong with me. I just needed to change my perspective, give my body a voice and start moving again.

I always hated exercising in the morning, so I would go after work, but then it got too late. I found some Pilates exercises worked well for me in the morning and a shorter workout in the evening. It didn't matter what it was at the end of the day, so long as my body was moving.

But I didn't start there wisely. Right in the beginning, I decided to go full-on with gym-style workouts and successfully burned out my body in a very short time. I was trying so hard to get fit, trying so hard to be well, that I was ignoring what was actually happening in my thoughts and in my body.

I learned that acknowledging what feels wrong—acknowledging the illness in the body rather than boldly trying to ignore it or shove it out of existence—is required before any shift towards complete wellness can be achieved.

I had a weak immune system, a weak digestive system, weak muscles in my neck, shoulders, and hips, and a wild skin condition on my feet. For the most part, I could hide this from everyone I knew, but out of the public eye, I was suffering. I didn't realize how often I sat during the day; despite believing I led a busy lifestyle. I didn't realize how poor my diet had become.

Once I began to truly acknowledge these realities, I started with my mental health, bringing my thoughts into alignment. Then I worked in small increments on strengthening different parts of my physical body.

Rediscovering Joy and Connection

Having fun was also something that became completely foreign to me. I didn't go out anymore and when I thought of all the things I used to do for fun, I no longer wanted to do those things. I didn't want to try new things and I did not want to meet new people. But just by going out of the house for a walk, I ended up meeting new friends. I started volunteering meeting more new people, we even had Christmas in July which was so much fun. Very slowly, I began getting out again and finding enjoyment in new activities.

Movement became my bridge back to the world. When we move, we naturally encounter others—fellow walkers on trails, people in fitness classes, volunteers at community events. There's something about the shared experience of physical activity that breaks down barriers and creates natural connections. We're all just bodies in motion, working toward feeling better, and that common ground can be the foundation for meaningful friendships.

As I reconnected with movement and began building new relationships, I realized there was another fundamental aspect of my body's function I had completely lost touch with—my breath.

Breath: Reclaiming Your Life Force

When I first discovered breathwork, it felt extreme and dizzying. I had to be very gentle with my body in rediscovering my breath. My body had been operating in survival mode for so long that conscious, deep breathing felt foreign and overwhelming. The irony is profound: our bodies instinctively know how to breathe, yet after prolonged exposure to the stress of domestic violence, we literally forget how to breathe properly.

When survival becomes our only focus, breath becomes one of the casualties. Our nervous system remains on high alert, constantly scanning for danger, bracing for the next threat. In this heightened state, our breath becomes a casualty of survival. We hold our breath when we hear footsteps approaching. We take shallow, rapid breaths from our chest rather than deep, nourishing breaths from our belly. We might even unconsciously restrict our breathing—making ourselves smaller, quieter, less noticeable.

During moments of acute stress or threat, the impact on our breath becomes even more pronounced. When fear grips us, our breathing may become rapid and shallow, or we might find ourselves holding our breath entirely without realizing it. The body tightens, the chest constricts, and oxygen struggles to reach where it's needed most. This restricted breathing perpetuates the cycle of fear and anxiety, keeping our nervous system locked in that fight-or-flight response.

Even after we've left the situation, our bodies can remain trapped in this pattern. The nervous system and breath continue operating as if danger is still present, still imminent. This is the body's way of trying to protect us, but it leaves us exhausted, disconnected, and unable to fully inhabit our own lives. When we breathe shallowly and rapidly, our brain and body are starved of the oxygen they desperately need to function optimally.

This oxygen deprivation creates a fog—a mental cloudiness that makes it difficult to think clearly, make decisions, or even remember simple things. We may find ourselves forgetting appointments, struggling to concentrate on conversations, or feeling like we're moving through life in a daze. I would describe this as feeling like I had a wet towel wrapped around my head with two tiny eyes holes cut out. The exhaustion isn't just physical; it's cognitive and emotional too. Our capacity for joy, creativity, and clear thinking becomes severely diminished when our most basic life force—our breath—remains constricted.

Reclaiming our breath is reclaiming our life force. It is one of the most powerful steps toward healing and becoming truly vibrant again.

I chose not to follow any single "breathwork" method. In my experience, there were too many variables, and most techniques left me dizzy, feeling like I would lose consciousness. Some were intense and even a little scary! However, from studying those various techniques, I did learn the importance of making conscious breath practice part of my daily life.

What I found unhelpful was when people would simply tell me to "just breathe" without offering any real direction or information. Once, in an office somewhere, someone showed me a technique: "Now just take a breath up into the left-hand corner of the room. Breathe out, and now take a breath into the right-hand corner of the room..." This went nowhere for me. Rather than calming me, it left me feeling hopeless, angry, stuck, and frustrated.

The breath alone wasn't my saviour. It was a culmination of small changes, gentle exercises, and some brain training that brought my body back to a state of well-being—it was the beginning of my Vibrant! I became dedicated to whole wellness in body and mind.

Movement and breath work together, but there's a third element that's equally essential to switching off that sympathetic nervous system and allowing true healing to occur: the practice of genuine relaxation.

The Power of Relaxation: Teaching Your Body It's Safe

One of the most challenging aspects of healing from domestic violence is learning to truly relax. When your body has spent months or years in a constant state of alert, relaxation doesn't come naturally—it has to be relearned. This isn't laziness or "doing nothing". Relaxation is an active practice of teaching your nervous system that it's safe to let down its guard.

True relaxation is the gateway to activating your parasympathetic nervous system—that essential "rest and digest" mode where healing actually occurs. Without periods of genuine relaxation, your body cannot repair damaged tissues, regulate hormones properly, strengthen your immune system, or process and integrate the trauma you've experienced. Your body literally needs permission to stop being on guard, and relaxation is how you give that permission.

I discovered that relaxation came in many forms, and different approaches worked for different days and different needs. Sometimes it was simply lying down in the afternoon sun, feeling the warmth on my skin and allowing my muscles to soften into the ground beneath me. Other times it was a warm bath where I consciously released tension from each part of my body. I enjoyed the process of Yoga Nidra and I learned that relaxation could be gentle stretching, listening to calming music, sitting quietly with a cup of tea, or even just sitting still and watching clouds move across the sky.

What made these moments truly restorative wasn't just the physical stillness—it was the mental permission I gave myself to rest without guilt. For so long, I had believed that rest meant weakness, that I had to be constantly doing something to prove my worth or ensure my safety. Learning that rest was actually a productive part of healing, not a waste of time, changed everything.

The practice of relaxation taught my body that danger had passed. Each time I consciously relaxed, I was sending a message to my nervous system: "We are safe now. You can rest. You don't need to protect us right now". Over time, these moments of intentional relaxation began to reprogram my body's default state. The hypervigilance gradually loosened its grip.

I also learned that relaxation didn't mean forcing myself to be still when my body was buzzing with nervous energy. Sometimes the path to relaxation was through gentle movement first—a slow walk, some stretching, or rhythmic activities that helped discharge the excess stress hormones before true rest could settle in.

The key was consistency and compassion. Even five minutes of genuine relaxation daily made a difference. I stopped waiting for the "right time" or until I had "earned" rest. Relaxation became a non-negotiable part of my healing practice, as essential as eating or breathing. I began to learn to use this powerful tool in between body movement to create balance for myself.

I noticed there were times it was difficult to relax and came to the realisation it had to do with what I was feeding my body—not just with food, but with every form of energy I was consuming.

What Goes In: Nourishing Your Body and Soul

Being aware of what goes into the body sounds easy, but there is so much information in the world about nutrition that without becoming a nutritionist, it's difficult territory to navigate. Again, there were programs and diets—do this for stress relief, eat that for energy, 122 healthy recipes, 14 steps to wellness. The list goes on.

What I've come to understand is that nutrition is deeply personal. What nourishes one woman's body may not work for another. Our bodies have been through different traumas, carry different sensitivities, and have different needs. There is no one-size-fits-all approach to healing and well-being through food. But it is a super important part of the after DV healing process. It is part of the big picture, part of the new identity, part of you being your true Divine, Intelligent, Vibrant and Authentic new self.

In addition to food, other energies we put into our bodies have a profound effect on how our bodies react and operate. Everything we consume becomes energy—the food we eat, the media we watch, the thoughts we dwell on, the environments we allow ourselves to inhabit.

I'd always thought I had been good to my body. I ate foods that were good for my body, fresh fruits and vegies mostly, legumes and fish. I exercised, looked after myself, didn't drink alcohol, didn't smoke, didn't do drugs. And yet here I was in a state of dis-ease. What I wasn't realizing was what I was feeding myself environmentally. Those were my poisons, my toxins.

Allowing and enabling a perpetrator of DV to disrespect and harm my body—that was what I was feeding myself. The shows I was watching on TV, many with elements of violence—that was what I was feeding my body. Watching the news, absorbing stories of crimes and tragedy—that's what I was feeding my body.

In addition to these toxins, any time I spoke negatively about the DV experience, the perpetrator or anyone else who I perceived had wronged or harmed me, I was in effect attacking them, pouring all that negative energy and disdain onto them—and hence feeding that to myself too. You cannot attack another person without attacking yourself. You cannot hurt another person without hurting yourself. I realised I was not at peace, and I was adding even more negative energy to my body.

Buddhist teachings recognize that violence isn't limited to physical acts—it includes harmful speech and even negative thoughts directed toward another person. This understanding opened my eyes to how I was continuing to harm myself long after leaving the abusive situation. It was a difficult moment for me to admit and took a little personal courage!

But it didn't stop there. I was also attacking my own body with my thoughts and feelings about it and about myself..

I looked in the mirror and could only see an unattractive, sad, broken person. I could see every perceived fault. My focus became fixated on what was wrong with my body. I was attacking it with my thoughts, so frustrated with my feet that I obsessed over the dis-ease there. Instead of being kind, gentle, and loving to my body, I was scratching, scraping, soaking, rubbing creams on it, taking medications to try and mask the pain. It was an endless cycle.

All of this was manifesting in my body as dis-ease. That was a heavy wake-up call for me, but very enlightening at the same time.

Living Vibrant: Feeling Into What Feels Good

My journey back to vibrant health wasn't a straight line with clear steps—it was an intertwined path where everything connected to everything else. Movement helped my breath, breath calmed my nervous system, a calmer nervous system improved my digestion, better digestion gave me energy to move. It was all woven together, each element supporting the others.

In the beginning, I felt desperate to fix myself. I threw everything at the problem—intense workouts, strict regimens, attempting to force my body back into health. But that desperation came from a fundamental misunderstanding: I wasn't broken. My body and mind had adopted life-saving techniques during the domestic violence—techniques that had kept me safe but had become unhealthy patterns once I actually was safe. I didn't need fixing. I needed gentle guidance back to my natural state of being.

For a long time, it felt like a careful balancing act. Some days I managed it well, other days everything felt like too much. But gradually, almost without noticing, the practices became small habits woven into the fabric of my daily life. Exercise wasn't a task I had to force myself to do—it became something I just did, as natural and automatic as cleaning my teeth. Conscious breathing became a reflex rather than a deliberate practice. Choosing nourishing foods felt less like discipline and more like self-love. Relaxation stopped feeling like giving up and started feeling like coming home to myself.

It was really just a matter of guiding myself—my attention and my thoughts—back to being. Back to the natural state my body had always known before survival mode took over.

The transformation didn't happen overnight, but one day I realized I wasn't thinking about these practices anymore—I was simply living them. My body had remembered what vibrant felt like, and now it naturally gravitated toward the things that kept me there

Here's how I approach my Vibrant now: I feel into what feels good. Genuinely. Without tricking myself into anything, without telling myself little untruths, without being apologetic, and without justifying or judging myself.

Feel what feels good. You don't need to find what feels good, just feel into it. Soften and feel. When a person extends an invitation, feel into it. If it feels good, go with it. If not, just say so. Thanks for asking, but that won't work for me at this time. This will work with anything and everything as you listen to your inner guidance and wisdom. When choosing food, feel into it. Does this food feel good for me right now? The feeling will always tell you; you just need to tune in and listen and feel. Can you remember a time when you really didn't want to do something, but did it anyway? Through the DV journey, this was solely for your survival, but outside of DV, feeling into how you feel about something (or someone) is a life changing technique.

The vibrant life isn't just about having energy—it's about feeling alive in your own skin, connected to your strength, and open to the joy that comes from a body that moves with freedom and grace. It's about a nervous system that knows it's safe, a breath that flows freely, muscles that move with ease, and a spirit that recognizes rest as sacred. It's about nourishing yourself with food, thoughts, and experiences that honour the divine temple your body truly is.

You are not broken. You are remembering. You are becoming vibrant again.

Part three tools & practices

Your body holds the wisdom of your healing. After trauma, we often disconnect from our physical selves as a protective mechanism. Physical healing creates a cascade of renewal that touches every aspect of your being. When you nourish your body, you're not just feeding cells - you're feeding your spirit. When you move your body, you're not just building strength - you're releasing trapped emotions and creating space for joy. When you rest your body, you're not just recovering - you're allowing your nervous system to remember what safety feels like.

True vibrancy emerges when we reunite mind, body, and spirit - when we remember that we are not broken, but beautifully resilient beings ready to thrive again. With the body mind and soul united once again you are no longer fragmented by trauma but functioning as the unified, powerful system you were meant to be living your vibrant self.

The A+ instant reset

This simple technique is powerful in any moment of high emotion, fear or illness. Every time something comes up in your body feel into it and allow it to release so you can experience calm and ease and allow something different.

Use in moments of exploration, overwhelm, fear, not knowing what to do, anxiety, physical illness.

1. **Acknowledge** - You are aware that you are feeling off, feeling fear or feeling dis-ease in your body. Acknowledge that. Listen to the body for a moment. Feel into the emotions. Allow the feelings to be there, no matter how intense. Don't be afraid if they intensify while you are acknowledging them. Tell your body "I am aware, I feel you body, thank you body for protecting me, thank you for this communication". Rate the discomfort on a scale of 1 – 10 and be totally ok with it.
2. **Air** – Your reminder to breathe into it. Regardless of if you feel heightened or you feel like you don't need to calm down, take a moment to relax into your current feeling. It's ok that I am feeling this. It's ok that I am here now with this happening. Breathe in through the nose for 5 seconds, pause, breathe out like you are gently blowing a candle out for 7-8 seconds. Pause your breath before breathing in again. Breath deep into the

belly allowing it to expand and allow the belly to sink in as your release the breath. Do this 3 times.
3. **Allow** – When you acknowledge the feelings in your body (step 1) this allows for a transmutation of the energy. Rather than resisting, shoving it down, ignoring it, you acknowledge it to allow the shift. By breathing (Step 2) you have calmed your nervous system. From this place of acknowledgement and calm, you can now allow something different. There are two ways to do this.

Ask; how does it get better than this? what would it take for...? what is possible here?

Or,

Affirm; I am allowing peace in my body now, I am allowing something new, I choose to feel calm, I am stronger than this moment, I am moving through this.

Quick version of The A+ instant reset.

A – Acknowledge the feelings. I am feeling _____ in my body.

A – Air – your reminder to breathe. In for five, out for eight, three times.

A – Allow something different using Ask or Affirm – What's the best that can happen? I am moving through this experience.

Mirror Practice

The first time I decided to speak to myself in the mirror, I took one look at the broken lady in the reflection, and I cried and cried. I called it ugly cry, cos it sure wasn't pretty! It was so difficult, I felt even less beautiful seeing my ugly cry and no words would come out. When I had composed myself, I started by saying "Hi", and then looking away.

Now I look in the mirror at home, the reflection of the car door, shop windows or mirrors and I can almost give my reflection a high five. I say "Hi beautiful", and I can usually feel amazing! This exercise is powerful and works. Of course everyone has off days, me too, but this one is good to keep practicing.

Stand in front of a mirror and speak to yourself as you would to a beloved friend. Start with simple affirmations like "Hello (your name), you are worthy".

This can be a little confronting if you haven't done it before. And as with any affirmation, if it doesn't ring true, try softening it a little. Instead of going straight for "Hello (your name), I love you and admire you. You are strong and Beautiful!", maybe start gently "Hello (your name), I see you".

It is important not to resist the resistance. Gently notice what resistance comes up, this shows you where your vibration needs healing attention. If you are struggling with telling yourself you are beautiful, and there is a tightening in the body, just look at yourself and say "It's ok that I feel this way". Start with a smaller part of the body to love and appreciate that doesn't have an emotional charge. It could be that your hair looks nice today. "Hello (your name), your hair looks lovely today".

As you progress and become more comfortable, you can give your reflection, your divine self, reminders. "Hi beautiful, remember you are divine, and I love you". Use some of your favourite "I am" affirmations. There is a list of affirmations in the *Additional Tools & Practices* section at the back of this book. Choose the ones that fit you or tweak them slightly.

Each time you pass your reflection, get into the habit of quickly thinking to yourself or saying out loud, "hello lovely!" or something nice that you might say when you see someone you love.

Nourishing the Temple

I didn't realize it, but for a long time I was using convenience foods because it was something I didn't need to think about. Cooking a nutritious meal for myself was not at the forefront of my mind. Staying out of danger was.

As you reclaim your life and step into vibrancy, nourishing your body becomes an act of self-love and self-respect. This isn't about perfection or strict diets—it's about becoming aware of what you're putting into your body and learning to listen to what it truly needs.

Here are a few simple practices to begin:

1. Take Stock Do an honest inventory of your pantry and fridge. How much processed food are you using? No judgment here—just awareness. When you're ready, try switching one or two processed foods for natural alternatives. Small steps create lasting change.

2. Speak to Your Body Yes! Your body will give you an indication of what foods you need when you listen to it. Before you eat something, pause and ask yourself: *"Is this food right for me in this moment?"* Notice how your body responds. Does it feel expansive and energized, or heavy and resistant? Your body has wisdom—learn to trust it.

This practice isn't about restriction; it's about connection. When you nourish your body with intention, you're cultivating vitality, strength, and vibrance.

3. Mindful eating

Transform eating from a rushed necessity into a nurturing ritual. Even if it's just five minutes, sit down without distractions—no phone, no television, no multitasking. Take a breath before you begin. Notice the colours, textures, and aromas of your food. As you eat, chew slowly and be present with each bite.

This simple act of mindful eating honours your body and reinforces that you are worthy of this time, this nourishment, this care. It shifts eating from autopilot to intention—and that's where true vibrance begins.

Movement Practice

Your body was designed to move, and movement is medicine for both body and mind. When we've been in survival mode, our bodies can hold tension, stress, and stagnant energy. Movement helps release what no longer serves us and creates space for vitality to flow.

You don't need a gym membership or hours of free time. You just need to begin where you are, with what you have.

Here are two simple practices to bring movement into your day:

Morning Stretch and Breathe - Before you even get out of bed, take a moment to stretch your body. Reach your arms overhead, point and flex your feet, roll your shoulders, gentle twist your spine. Take three deep breaths as you move. This signals to your body that it's safe, it's supported, and a new day has begun. Even two minutes makes a difference.

Dance Break - Put on a song you love—something that makes you want to move—and let your body respond however it wants to. Shake, sway, jump, spin, or simply move your arms. There's no right or wrong way. This isn't exercise; it's expression. It releases stuck energy, lifts your mood, and reminds you that your body is yours to enjoy.

Integrate movement into your day - Try 10 squats, while you are brushing your teeth, touch your toes 10 times before bed and when you get up, reach your hands above your head towards the ceiling 10 times when you cook that nutritional meal! Knees to chest when you walk to the car, or 10 wall push ups in the toilet! Take 5 minutes to take a short walk. Walk barefoot if you can on the grass or in the sand. Adding a little conscious movement to your day inspires more movement and creates great habits.

Movement doesn't have to be complicated. It just needs to happen. Every time you move with intention, you're creating strength, freedom, and vibrancy. As you get started with these simple exercises and feel that you want to do more, check out some yoga flow, palates or qi gong exercises. I recommend finding professional teachers who often share free content, no social media reels here!!

Part 4 – I AM AUTHENIC

Honouring our true voice and desires without fear or apology.

For the longest time, "authentic" was just a word I'd see on Italian recipes—it held no meaning for me beyond that. After my DV experience, I couldn't recognize myself in the mirror or imagine what I wanted from life anymore. The future I'd once envisioned had vanished, leaving me directionless and without purpose. This experience felt like a devastating punch to the gut that knocked the wind out of my sails, leaving me feeling useless, hopeless, and utterly lost. I couldn't remember what I was good at, who I'd been before it all happened or where my joy was.

I felt like a fraud among the people I interacted with, always putting on the happy face and smile and appearing as though I was doing fine. All the while feeling inadequate and diminished in their company. I remembered back to all the times the perpetrator in my life had said "I'll make sure you are nothing but an empty shell", and I felt like he had won on that point. I felt like an empty shell. No worth, no direction, no idea.

I learned very quickly that discovering my authentic self was not something I could jump onto the internet to find. I did actually search for "how to find my authentic self" and came up with such a wormhole of nonsense and nothing that resonated with me, written by psychologists and others who I am certain had not been through the experience of domestic violence. None of them made sense to me, it seemed there was so much to explore and I didn't have a clue where to start.

I decided to try and discover my authentic self, who I was, myself!

Who am I? The most frustrating question
Before I could even begin to discover *who* I was, I had to acknowledge that uncomfortable truth: I had no idea anymore. Perhaps the most disorienting part of this journey was the growing awareness that years of hypervigilance, people-pleasing, and survival strategies had created layers upon layers of defences until I felt like a stranger to myself. I would catch glimpses of my reflection and wonder, "Who is this person?". The woman staring back seemed like someone I should recognize yet felt like a complete stranger. She was hollow, a fraction of herself.

I kept hearing the spiritual messages from teachers calm, serene, sitting in their peaceful spaces in carefully edited YouTube videos or on masterclasses tell me to simply ask myself "Who am I?". They made it sound like a gateway, as if asking this profound question would unlock some mystical breakthrough, and a sudden clarity that would illuminate everything. But for me? It felt utterly useless. I tried it. The question just hung there in the air, unanswered and frustrating. The roaring sound of crickets or just a deafening silence. Who am I? I don't know! That's the whole problem! It wasn't a gateway for me; it felt like hitting a brick wall over and over again—like repeatedly face-planting into a glass window right next to the automatic opening door.

So, I started asking myself different questions—more doable questions that didn't require some mystical breakthrough to answer. What did I really want in life? Where was my ideal place to live? Did I genuinely want to be in a relationship, or had I simply absorbed society's expectations of what I was supposed to want? What made me feel alive rather than just safe? The deeper I looked, the more I realised that many of my personality traits, opinions, and even interests had been shaped by society and survival rather than genuine authentic choice. The wonderful thing about questions, is they open up possibility.

But in exploring these questions, the uncomfortable truth was that I felt utterly inauthentic in my own skin. I had become so skilled at staying small, not speaking my truth, reading rooms, anticipating needs, and adapting to keep peace that I had lost touch with my own inner compass. Even in safety, I found myself automatically shifting into whatever version of myself seemed most socially acceptable. Although the physical threat was gone, the learned behaviours persisted. I began to notice myself behaving one way with a certain group of people and another way with different people. It was exhausting—and deeply lonely—to realise I had been performing my own life rather than living it.

This recognition, while painful, became a crucial starting point. I couldn't return to an authentic self I had never fully known. Instead, I had to give myself permission to discover who I was from scratch, approaching myself with the curiosity I might show a new friend. New questions continued to emerge. "Who am I right now?" and "Who am I becoming right now?". This journey of discovery required me to examine not just who I was now, but how and why I'd learned to hide myself in the first place. It would prove to give me a direction, and that was what I needed.

Hiding behind a persona

As I began this journey of self-discovery, I had to confront how deeply the pattern of hiding myself ran. DV causes us to create a false identity based on our need to survive. When we're living in an abusive situation, our authentic self becomes a luxury we can't afford. Every fibre of our being shifts into survival mode, and in that space, we learn to become whoever we need to be to stay safe, to keep the peace, or simply to make it through another day.

The person we become in an abusive relationship isn't really us—it's a carefully constructed survival persona. We learn to read micro-expressions, to anticipate moods before they shift, to make ourselves smaller when needed or invisible when it serves us. We become master shapeshifters, morphing into whatever version of ourselves causes the least conflict.

This survival identity might look like the woman who never expresses an opinion or preference, because having an opinion or preferences triggered rage. Or the one who became hypervigilant, always scanning for danger, always ready to flee or fight. Perhaps we became the peacekeeper, taking responsibility for everyone else's emotions, or the perfectionist, believing that if we could just be good enough, smart enough, quiet enough, the abuse would stop. I had learned in the DV environment to hide myself for my own safety, but this pattern went much deeper than I initially realized.

As I continued to explore this idea, I realized this pattern of hiding myself started long before domestic violence entered my life. Beyond the survival instincts that DV carved into me, I began recognizing a much longer pattern of hiding who I truly was. Childhood memories surfaced, countless moments when being authentically me simply wasn't acceptable. I was too old for certain games, too young for others, too smart to act "that way." At school, my body shape, music taste, and hobbies became targets for ridicule. Each instance was a small but persistent message: your authentic self isn't accepted here. In addition, I was taught to not use my voice, my opinion didn't matter. I was taught to be kind and considerate to others, putting their own needs before my own, believing there was a virtue in that. I was shamed for voicing my needs and expressing my choices.

These weren't isolated incidents but a continuous stream of psychological and social conditioning that taught me to suppress my true nature and conform to whatever version of myself others found acceptable. Society had already been teaching me what was "appropriate" for a girl, for a woman—how to dress, how to speak, what behaviours were ladylike, what ambitions were realistic. I was told in high school being an author is not a real job, so my dreams were dismissed. The unspoken rules were everywhere: don't be too loud, don't be too opinionated, don't be too ambitious, don't take up too much space. Be agreeable. Be pleasant. Be helpful. Make others comfortable, even at the expense of our own comfort.

I learned early that creating a persona wasn't just about physical survival—it was about navigating a world that had very specific expectations about who I should be. It was about fitting into boxes that society had pre-constructed: the good daughter, the supportive friend, the accommodating colleague, the selfless mother, the good wife. These roles came with scripts, and deviating from those scripts often meant judgment, criticism, or social exclusion. The persona became my way of feeling safe in social situations, of being accepted, of avoiding the pain of rejection, ridicule, or being labelled as "difficult," "too much," or "not enough."

Long before domestic violence entered my life, I had already taken on a persona, to hide my genuine interests and reactions, to edit my opinions to match the room, to shrink myself down to fit into spaces that were never designed for the real me. That persona became my protection not just from abuse, but from the everyday wounds of being judged, criticized, or dismissed simply for being authentically myself in a world that preferred women to be palatable and predictable.

She's Been There All Along

But here's the truth I discovered: underneath all those survival strategies, our authentic self has been waiting. She's been there all along, perhaps pushed so far down that we can barely hear her whisper, but she's never left us. She's the part of us that knew something was wrong even when everyone else said we were overreacting. She's the spark that eventually gave us the strength to leave, even when leaving felt impossible.

The journey back to authenticity after abuse is about gently peeling away these survival identities and asking ourselves: "Who am I when I'm not afraid? Who am I when I don't have to manage someone else's emotions? Who am I when I'm not walking on eggshells?".

The answers might surprise us. We might discover we're naturally bold, naturally creative, naturally opinionated. We might find that we love things we convinced ourselves we hated, or that we have dreams we buried so deep we forgot they existed.

This isn't about blame or shame—those survival identities saved our lives. Honour them for what they did, thank them for keeping us safe, and then gently let them know they can rest now. We're safe enough to be real now. We're safe enough to be ourselves.

Dealing with Doubt and Shame

Knowing my authentic self was there, waiting beneath all those layers of protection, didn't automatically make her easy to access. Between recognizing she existed and actually connecting with her stood two formidable gatekeepers: doubt and shame. These twin forces worked in tandem, creating a fortress around my authentic self that felt nearly impossible to breach.

The Voice of Doubt

The road to authenticity felt impossibly long, stretching out before me like a highway riddled with a million potholes—and doubt was by far the deepest crater of them all. The doubt came in relentless waves: "What should I do with my life? Can I actually do this? Who am I to be this, want this, do this? I'll never be strong enough, smart enough, worthy enough". The voice of doubt was particularly cruel because it masqueraded as logic, whispering seemingly reasonable arguments for why I should just give up and settle for the familiar discomfort of inauthenticity.

What made doubt so insidious was how it fed on the very uncertainty that authentic living requires. To discover who we truly are, we must be willing to not know—to sit in the uncomfortable space between who we've been and who we're becoming. Doubt exploited this vulnerability, turning every moment of uncertainty into evidence of failure. It convinced me that "real" people had their lives figured out, that authenticity should feel clear and confident, not messy and questioning.

For me, there was an almost tangible tension between wanting growth and clinging to what was familiar—and this push-pull is such a universal part of the healing journey. Yet knowing this didn't make it any easier to step out of my comfort zone. My brain, with all its logical reasoning, kept insisting I was safer staying exactly where I was. The familiar pain felt manageable; the unknown felt terrifying.

The Weight of Shame

Working alongside doubt was an even heavier burden: shame. While doubt questioned my capabilities, shame attacked my very worth. I suffered the embarrassment that came with anyone knowing my story. This was a two-way street where I felt like I needed to say small parts of what had happened so people understood my situation and why I wasn't thriving, why I needed help, why I wasn't quite as good as they were, while trying to balance the feeling of shame that came with it.

Shame operates differently from guilt in the aftermath of abuse. While guilt says, "I did something wrong", shame whispers something far more insidious: "I am wrong". For 'survivors' of domestic violence, shame becomes a heavy cloak that distorts how we see ourselves. It convinces us that the abuse happened because of some fundamental flaw in our being—that we were too much or not enough, too weak for staying or too damaged for leaving. This shame often feels like a secret we must hide, even after we've escaped the relationship. It makes us question our judgment, our worth, and our right to move forward unburdened.

The Destructive Dance

What makes this combination of doubt and shame so destructive is how they reinforce each other, creating a vicious cycle. Shame tells us we're fundamentally flawed, and doubt uses that belief as evidence that we'll never succeed in changing. Doubt questions our ability to heal, and shame whispers that we don't deserve healing anyway. Together, they force us to live behind a veil.

When we carry shame, we cannot show up as our authentic selves—instead, we perform a version of ourselves we think is acceptable, lovable, or believable. We edit our stories, minimize our experiences, and hide parts of ourselves. Shame tells us that if people knew the truth—about what we endured, what we tolerated, or who we became during the abuse—they would judge us as harshly as we judge ourselves. And doubt confirms this fear, insisting that we're not strong enough, not worthy enough, not enough period, to move beyond it.

So, we stay small, stay quiet, and stay hidden. We doubt our ability to change and feel ashamed of who we are. The result? We remain trapped in a performance, disconnected from the authentic self who has been patiently waiting for us all along.

Breaking Through

But here's what I began to understand: doubt wasn't my enemy—it was actually a sign that I was finally asking the right questions. The fact that I was questioning everything meant I was no longer accepting the default programming that trauma had installed. Doubt, I realized, was often authenticity trying to break through the noise. The key wasn't eliminating doubt but learning to hear the quiet voice of truth beneath its clamour, trusting that the answers would emerge not through force, but through patient, compassionate self-discovery.

And shame? Shame thrived in secrecy and silence, just like DV. The moment I began to speak my truth—first to myself, then to trusted others—shame began to lose its grip. I discovered that shame couldn't survive in the light of honest acknowledgment and compassion. When I stopped judging myself so harshly and started treating myself with the same kindness I'd offer a dear friend, shame's power diminished, and so did the power that DV had over me.

Living authentically requires the opposite of what doubt and shame demand: it asks us to show up fully, messily, truthfully. The path from 'survivor' to DIVA isn't about becoming perfect or polished—it's about recognizing doubt as a sign of growth rather than failure and shedding the shame that keeps us performing so we can finally allow ourselves to simply be. When we release shame and work through doubt with self-compassion, we reclaim the right to exist as our whole, unedited selves.

The tools and techniques in each section of this book will help you release shame and work through doubt, including an EFT tapping exercise at the end of this part. But even as I worked to release these twin barriers and recognize the veil I'd been wearing, there was another formidable obstacle blocking my path to authenticity: my nervous system itself was working against me.

Breaking Free from Survival Mode

Even as I worked to release shame and recognize the veil I'd been wearing, there was another formidable obstacle blocking my path to authenticity: my nervous system itself was working against me.

Fight, flight, or freeze—these had become my default responses to every challenge life threw at me. Escaping the domestic violence environment felt like jumping into the fire from the frying pan. I had traded one set of survival-threatening circumstances for another, and my nervous system hadn't received the memo that I was finally safe.

Even as I asked the right questions and searched for answers, I remained trapped in fight-flight-freeze mode. This hypervigilant state made rediscovering my authentic self nearly impossible. How could I connect with who I truly was when my body and mind were constantly scanning for the next threat?

The cruel irony was clear: one of the greatest gifts of reclaiming authenticity is learning to see challenges as part of life's natural rhythm rather than existential threats. But here lay my catch-22—I needed a different perspective to move forward, yet my trauma-activated nervous system distorted my vision like a funhouse mirror.

Every thought spiralled toward worst-case scenarios. I could see my money running out with crystal clarity but couldn't envision it flowing back in. I could see the worst happening, people treating me badly and not see anyone as friend. I remained stuck in the problems rather than seeing challenges as potential fuel for growth. My survival brain simply couldn't access the creative, solution-focused thinking that my authentic self possessed.

Understanding the Survival Response

When we've lived through trauma, particularly ongoing threats like domestic violence, our nervous system becomes hyper tuned to danger. The amygdala—our brain's alarm system—develops a hair trigger, flooding our system with stress hormones at the slightest perceived threat. This neurobiological response, while lifesaving in genuinely dangerous situations, can persist long after we've reached safety.

In this state, the part of the brain responsible for creative problem-solving, long-term planning, and accessing our deeper wisdom—goes offline. We're literally unable to think our way out of survival mode; we must regulate our nervous system first. Only then can we begin to distinguish between genuine threats and growth opportunities, clearing the path back to our authentic selves. Calming the nervous system became a foundational tool I still use today in moments of uncertainty or to keep me from falling back into reactive habits.

Focus

As I learned tools to regulate my survival response, I began to notice something incredible. The calmer and more centred I became, the more I began noticing where my attention went and where it needed to be. The hypervigilance had trained me to focus outward, constantly scanning for danger. Now I needed to turn that focus inward, toward discovery rather than protection.

One of the most persistent side effects of domestic violence is how it rewires our focus. While living with abuse, hypervigilance kept us alive—our brains learned that constantly scanning for danger, anticipating the next rage, and focusing on what could go wrong was essential for survival. This wasn't weakness; it was adaptation. But now, in safety, this survival mechanism becomes a prison of its own. When our attention remains locked on threat detection, we cannot turn inward to discover who we truly are. We're so busy monitoring external dangers—watching for red flags, bracing for disappointment, rehearsing worst-case scenarios—that we have no energy left to explore our own desires, dreams, and authentic nature. Our focus becomes entirely reactive rather than creative. It's fascinating that these two words are made of the same letters, just in a different order. In essence, we need to switch the arrangement of those letters within ourselves—to transform from reactive to creative.

To live outside of being reactive, we must consciously redirect our attention from what we fear to who we are. This means training ourselves to notice not just what could hurt us, but what brings us joy, what ignites our curiosity, what feels true in our bodies. Authentic living requires us to shift from a focus of protection to a focus of self-discovery. When we redirect our gaze inward with gentleness and curiosity, we finally create space to meet ourselves—not the version that learned to survive, but the woman who was always there beneath the armour, veils and personas just waiting to be known.

But redirecting that gaze inward, while essential, raised an immediate challenge: when I finally looked within, what—or who—was I actually looking for? After years of survival mode, hypervigilance, and performing for others, the landscape of my inner world felt unfamiliar, almost foreign. I'd spent so long scanning outward for danger that turning inward felt like entering uncharted territory. And yet, this was precisely where the answers lived.

The Challenge of Finding My Inner Voice

To find these answers, I needed to circle back to my original questions: Who am I becoming? What do I want? What does my life mean?

As I explored these questions more deeply, I came to an important realization. My answer to the big question, "who am I", would shift and evolve at different stages of my life—and that was okay, and perhaps the reason why I found it so incredibly difficult to ask in the beginning. But at the core, beneath all the changing circumstances and roles, there was something constant, me. The essence of my true self, my divine self, my inner wisdom and my inner voice.

Understanding that I had an inner voice was one thing; actually hearing it clearly enough to let it shine was something else altogether. And once I understood that, my purpose became beautifully simple: let that innerness shine.

Developing my intuition and listening to my divine self, became a part of the journey that I intensely disliked at first, but gradually began to embrace as I progressed. Intuition was challenging work! Inner voice? What inner voice? I couldn't distinguish between the whisper of wisdom and that other voice—the one that constantly encouraged me to stay in my lane, remain in my safe little box, and avoid any risks. Then there were all the external voices from others that had spent years diminishing me, their echoes still reverberating in my head long after I'd left those situations behind.

The cacophony was overwhelming. How was I supposed to hear my authentic inner guidance when so many competing voices were shouting for attention? It felt like trying to have a quiet conversation in the middle of a construction site.

My Authentic Self and Her Inner Wisdom

So, what exactly is inner knowing, intuition, and inner wisdom? Think of your inner wisdom as your soul's GPS—a navigation system that has access to information your logical mind hasn't consciously processed yet. Unlike the fear-based voice that keeps you small and safe, or the critical external voices you've internalized, your inner wisdom speaks with a different quality entirely.

As a child, I would talk to myself in times of fear, despair, or illness. I'd tell myself I was okay, I would tell my body it would get better and that I was safe. I was speaking to my own body and mind, and as a small child, I knew instinctively how to do this. As I grew up, other influences took over and I stopped listening to that voice.

At some point during the DV experience, in moments of utter despair, I began doing this again—but it wasn't until after leaving that I began to realize the power of it. Speaking to the mind and the body is incredibly powerful. The knowing has been here all along. The experience of DV forced me to listen to it again.

As I studied and read, I realized all of the authors, writers, and speakers had the same messages, just delivered in different ways. As their words sank in, I'd almost have an unfurling in my deepest memories of self and a whispering of *I know this*. This book is the same—hopefully inspiring your memory of your true self.

Recognizing the Authentic Voice

Inner wisdom doesn't shout; it whispers. It doesn't criticize; it guides. It doesn't create panic; it offers clarity, even when that clarity leads you toward uncertainty. This voice carries the accumulated wisdom of your experiences—not just your trauma, but your resilience, your survival, your moments of joy and connection. It knows things your conscious mind has forgotten: your preferences before they were shaped by survival, your dreams before they were dimmed by others' limitations, your strength before it was questioned by those who needed you to stay small.

One of the most challenging aspects of reclaiming authenticity was learning to distinguish this genuine inner voice from the internalized critic that had taken up permanent residence in my head. The abuser's voice—whether from a partner, family member, or toxic relationship—doesn't disappear when we physically leave. It sets up shop in our minds, disguised as our own thoughts, whispering the same diminishing messages: "You're too much", "You're not enough", "Who do you think you are?".

The authentic voice speaks differently. Where the critic tears down, the authentic voice builds understanding. Where the critic creates shame, the authentic voice offers compassion. The critic says "You always mess up"; the authentic voice says "That didn't work—what can I learn?". Learning to recognize this difference was like learning to distinguish between two radio stations playing at the same time. It took practice, patience, and a willingness to tune in more carefully.

Trusting the Illogical

The tricky part is that inner wisdom often feels illogical. It might suggest leaving the stable job, ending the comfortable but unfulfilling relationship, or pursuing the dream that seems impossible. It asks you to trust something you can't prove, to follow a path you can't fully see. But here's what I learned: that voice that encouraged me to leave, to heal, to write this book, to trust my own experience—that was inner wisdom. It had been there all along, patiently waiting for me to quiet the noise enough to finally hear it.

When I hear my inner wisdom, it feels like peace in my body. I relax, I smile, I know. The goal is to practice and practice so the normal response to any challenge is to hear the inner voice. To me, that's what being authentic is—having the ability to tune in to how something feels, to speak from the soul, hearing my inner voice, feeling my intuition. To say out loud, "that won't work for me" or "I would rather do..." or "yes, that sounds wonderful".

Asking Questions, Finding Answers

In my practice of hearing my inner voice and strengthening my intuition, I asked questions and wrote them down. The wonderful thing about a question is that you don't need the answer. This sounds counterintuitive, but the moment a question is asked, you can shift into the energy of the answer or the solution which is already available—you just haven't tuned into it yet. So, for me it really was all about fine-tuning the energy. Stepping out of the energy of doubt, stepping into the energy of focusing on what I wanted. Steering away from the energy of fear. Moving away from the energy of shame. Feeling into myself by asking. The interesting thing is the answer doesn't come instantly like a voice from above, but it comes in the form of a knowing, a feeling, a happening.

After acknowledging all the challenges—the guilt, shame, fear, doubt—it became easier to ask: who am I and why am I here? When I began to clear the hurdles that stood in the way of me becoming my authentic self, the energy was different. My energy was different. These were no longer loaded questions full of uncertainty, but pathways to possibility. What do I want? This was an interesting question in the beginning because I could immediately delve into what I didn't want. I was completely focused on everything I didn't want. What do I love? What do I love doing? Who am I when I am being my authentic self?

The Journey of Small Steps

Holistically, when we do the techniques and exercises, and then shift into asking the questions, we are moving that little compass point and gradually begin travelling in a new direction. The more we do it and the more comfortable we get with doing these exercises and practices, the easier it gets, and they become a part of our new habits. These new habits help form new beliefs and soon enough bigger changes in life become more evident. It can really be like looking down carefully at each footstep, then you look up and realize how far you have come. Like a little kid learning to ride a bike who is so focused on watching his feet on the pedals that he hasn't realized he has actually ridden a long way!

The fabulous part of being our authentic self is the alignment we feel when we are. When our thoughts, actions and words match our true desires and values, this alignment feels wonderful. We start to notice that things just "work out" or the day just flows. We say no when we want to, and something better shows up. We don't go out of obligation, but because we truly want to, or we don't go because we actually don't want to. We create space for life in this aligned state.

Self-Honouring vs. Selfishness

As I connected more with my inner wisdom and experienced moments of alignment, I felt as though I was becoming more of me. I was practicing the techniques and tools I had gathered to live more authentically in my daily life. I was learning more and really enjoying the curiosity I was experiencing. Often within learning journeys, there is an unlearning process. For me, that meant unlearning patterns and habits that had kept me trapped for years.

I had to unlearn the toxic messaging that equated self-care with selfishness. There's a profound difference between healthy self-honouring and actual selfishness. Selfishness takes without regard for others' wellbeing. Self-honouring recognizes that I can't give what I don't have, that I can't love others authentically if I'm constantly betraying myself.

Self-honouring means saying no when I mean no, asking for what I need, and setting boundaries that protect my energy and wellbeing. It means recognizing that my needs matter just as much as everyone else's—not more, but certainly not less. This wasn't selfish; it was essential. I couldn't be genuinely present for others when I was constantly abandoning myself.

The Dishonesty of People-Pleasing

Perhaps the most uncomfortable realization was that I was people-pleasing, and not just within the DV environment but in other situations as well. It was actually a form of dishonesty. When I said yes because I felt like I had to, but wanted to say no. When I agreed to something to avoid conflict or a blow up, I was living a lie. But people pleasing is something we often have instilled in us from an early age to make our parents happy or to be a good girl, or to make friends in primary school, or to get a promotion at work. Nothing authentic here, just a lie as we do what we think we have to do to keep the peace, have people like us or to benefit in some way.

In my life, people-pleasing promised safety and acceptance, in the DV journey, mostly safety. But it delivered neither. Instead, I had co-created difficult and uncomfortable (and in some instances unsafe) situations for myself and often I didn't even realise I was people-pleasing.

Setting Boundaries

Boundaries are fundamentally about honouring ourselves, our true voice and desires without fear or apology. They are one of the most profound acts of self-love we can practice. When we set boundaries, we are saying to ourselves and to the world: I matter. My needs are valid. My wellbeing is non-negotiable.

Boundaries are about knowing and communicating your limits. Not just knowing what is acceptable to you, but actively raising your level of what you accept. This shift is transformative. For so long, you may have accepted treatment, situations, or dynamics that diminished you. Setting boundaries means recognizing that you deserve better and being willing to enforce that truth.

Healthy boundaries help you honour your own needs and values, and they create the space for you to speak your truth even when it doesn't feel comfortable. They are not walls that shut people out; rather, they are clear guidelines that protect your energy, your peace, and your sense of self. They help you distinguish between what is yours to carry and what belongs to others. They allow you to say yes to what nurtures you and no to what depletes you.

Setting boundaries without fear requires courage, especially if you have been raised or conditioned to prioritize others' comfort or other needs over your own. It means learning to tolerate the discomfort that might arise when someone pushes back against your limits. Think about this—a moment of perceived discomfort now, or a lifetime of complete discomfort from not setting boundaries? The temporary awkwardness of asserting your needs is nothing compared to the long-term erosion of your wellbeing that comes from staying silent. It means trusting that people who truly respect you will honour your boundaries, and those who don't are revealing something important about their place in your life.

Self-love is the foundation of boundary-setting. When you love yourself, you naturally protect yourself. You stop over-explaining, over-apologizing, or seeking permission to take care of your own needs. You recognize that boundaries are not selfish—they are essential. They preserve your integrity and allow your relationships to be built on honesty rather than resentment or obligation.

Healthy boundaries look different for everyone, but they share common threads: clarity, consistency, and compassion. Clarity means knowing what you will and won't tolerate. Consistency means upholding those limits even when it's difficult. Compassion means extending grace to yourself as you learn this skill, and recognizing that boundary-setting is a practice, not a perfection.

Boundaries most definitely are the foundation for living authentically. Without them, we risk losing ourselves in the expectations, demands, and judgments of others. With them, we create the conditions for genuine connection, inner peace, and a life that truly reflects who we are. And here's what I discovered: when you commit to boundaries and authentic living, something remarkable happens in your relationships.

Living authentically acts as a natural filter in relationships. When I stopped contorting myself to fit others' expectations, something beautiful happened: the wrong people naturally drifted away, while the right people drew closer. Those who had been attracted to my compliance and availability became uncomfortable with my boundaries and self-respect. Meanwhile, people who valued authenticity, growth, and mutual respect began appearing in my life.

This wasn't always easy. Sometimes it meant letting go of friendships I'd invested years in building. But I learned that a friendship requiring me to betray myself wasn't actually a relationship worth having. Authentic living didn't guarantee that everyone would like me—but it guaranteed that those who did would be liking the real me.

Embracing Change

These revelations about authenticity became more than just personal insights—they became catalysts for profound transformation. Each moment of choosing honesty over harmony, boundaries over acceptance, and truth over comfort created ripples of change that extended far beyond my daily interactions. I began to see how every authentic choice, no matter how small, was actually an act of rebellion against the patterns that had kept me trapped, and how these accumulated moments of truth were quietly revolutionizing not just how I related to others, but how I related to life itself.

I went through the stage of being the victim—taking on the victim persona and fully inhabiting that identity. What happened to me was brutal, and I was indeed the victim of crime. That part was real and undeniable.

But that wasn't who I was. That wasn't the authentic me. It took time to rediscover myself, and a large part of what prolonged that journey was a fear I didn't even recognize at first: I was afraid of not being the victim anymore.

This subconscious fear came directly from being told over and over again that no one would believe me. It was one of the many threats that held me trapped in the DV environment. "People will think you're the crazy one", "You can't tell anyone—no one will believe you". It was all part of the carefully orchestrated control plan that holds victims firmly in a state of fear and as far away from their authentic selves as possible.

The thing about life is that things happen for a reason—to help us grow and expand, to offer more, to be more, and to become an active, bright part of all that is. When we encounter experiences that carry messages designed to help us explore and become more of ourselves, we often miss those messages entirely. This happens partly because we've been programmed from a very early age and have lost the ability to tune into the universal communications that come from our inner selves.

When we become skilled at ignoring these messages, they inevitably get louder. They keep amplifying until something catastrophic happens in our lives—because sometimes that's what it takes to finally get our attention.

In my life, this disconnection from my authentic self, festered over decades. I was receiving messages, but because I wasn't accustomed to tuning into the frequency of my true self, I simply wasn't hearing them. I had opportunities to expand and become more of myself early in childhood, but being ridiculed, told to shut up, to be seen and not heard, caused me to disconnect from the universe and my authentic self.

So, the messages got louder and louder, until I found myself in a position where I believed I would lose my life. That was the biggest wake-up call, the loudest message possible, that I wasn't living authentically as my true self.

My somewhat comical conversation with the universe went something like this:

"Gee Universe, I nearly died back there! What the hell. You are supposed to love and protect me".

"I do love you".

"But you nearly got me killed!".

"You weren't listening".

"I was!".

"You were not listening. I was messaging you".

"Well, I didn't get the messages".

"You got the last one...".

"Yes, lucky for that, or I would be dead by now—and no thanks to you".

"That was me literally shouting at you to listen to your inner self and live an authentic life".

"Oh, could you not have put it that simply before?".

"I did. You weren't listening".

In a sense I really felt as though the whole situation of living with DV was the biggest challenge of my life and through this experience I journeyed to find growth, peace and expansion in my life. While other people have equally painful and challenging life experiences, the invitation to change and to grow is the same. Being able to step completely away from the emotional turmoil, the pain and suffering and to be able to see this experience from a different perspective really did change my life. I began listening in to the whisper of intuition, the messages from the universe (or God) and ultimately the messages from my inner self, my own wisdom. I wondered through all of this if there really was a way of learning and expanding without the hurt and the discomfort, but that's also an invitation to look at hurt and suffering from a different perspective. Suffering, I found out, really is optional. When we learn to disconnect from the suffering with daily practices and new awareness, then it no longer exists. Wow, that's a relief and every time I remind myself "suffering is optional," it brings a smile to my face.

Resistance to Change and Challenges

Resistance is a natural protective response to pain, but it often keeps us trapped in the very suffering we're trying to escape. When we've experienced trauma, our instinct is to push away the difficult emotions, to numb ourselves, or to stay perpetually busy so we don't have to feel. But what we resist persists—it lives in our bodies, shapes our choices, and builds walls between us and our authentic selves.

The path back to yourself requires a different kind of courage: the courage to stop fighting your own experience. When you allow yourself to feel the grief, the anger, the fear—without judgment, without needing to fix it immediately—something remarkable happens. The energy moves through you rather than getting stuck. You discover that you're strong enough to hold your own pain, that feeling it won't destroy you. In this allowing, in this radical acceptance of what is, you reclaim the parts of yourself that went into hiding. You become whole again, not by erasing what happened, but by honouring your journey through it. Your authentic self isn't waiting on the other side of your pain—she emerges as you bravely walk through it.

The journey to authenticity isn't a destination you reach—it's a practice you return to, again and again. Some days you'll speak your truth with clarity and confidence. Other days you'll catch yourself slipping back into old patterns, saying yes when you mean no, shrinking to make others comfortable. And that's okay. This is what it means to be human, to be healing, to be growing.

What matters is that you keep choosing yourself. That you keep asking the questions, listening for your inner wisdom, and honouring the woman you're becoming. The veil you wore, the persona you created kept you alive, but they don't serve you anymore. Your authentic self—the one who's been waiting patiently beneath all those layers of protection—is ready to step into the light. She's been there all along, and now, finally, you're ready to meet her.

Living authentically after domestic violence isn't about becoming someone new. It's about remembering who you were before the world taught you to hide, and then becoming who you were always meant to be. It's about reclaiming your voice, your boundaries, your right to take up space in your own life. And when you do this—when you commit to showing up as your whole, unedited self—you don't just transform your own life, you become a beacon for others still finding their way home to themselves.

Part four tools & practices

Becoming authentic is a journey of rediscovery—peeling back the layers of survival personas and protective masks to reconnect with the wisdom that has been within you all along. You've learned that your inner knowing has been patiently waiting, that doubt can be released, and that living authentically means honouring your truth through boundaries and aligned action.

These practices aren't about perfection—they're about returning to yourself, again and again, with patience and self-compassion. Each time you use these tools, you're choosing authenticity and your genuine self over the persona that kept you safe but small.

Stillness meditation

No matter where you are, as long as it safe to do so, slow down, then pause, then stop all together.

Find a comfortable place to sit or stand to be still. Let the busy-ness of the world continue around you, but not touch you. Close your eyes and see yourself standing or sitting still.

See the world hurrying around you as though in fast forward and you suspended for a moment in this stillness.

Feel into peace. Where you are right now, peace is available to you, in this very moment.

Breathe slowly and deeply into the peace. Let yourself be still while surrounded by the hustle and bustle of activity swirling and moving around you. You remain untouchable, feeling into the peace.

Speak to your mind. "Thank you, mind, for protecting me. But in this moment, please be still. We are safe, I love you". "Peace is available to me in this moment".

Speak to your body. "Thank you, body, for supporting me. But in this moment, please be still. We are safe, I love you".

Stillness is your path to peace, intuition and divine guidance. Stillness inspires quiet in the moment. Stillness allows you to hear the messages you need. Remember to breathe in and out, slowly, deeply in the peace you have accessed now.

Focus on the feeling of peace and stillness while breathing slowly and deeply.

Take as long as you need, this meditation is powerful in short or in longer practices.

Reactive to Creative – bring your energy home

This is a simple exercise with remarkable results. We all know what it feels like to be reactive—the outburst, the sharp response, the overwhelming urge to release pent-up emotion. (Note: We're not talking about responding to emergencies here, this exercise focuses on unhelpful reactivity.)

Moving from Reactive to Creative might seem like a HUGE leap. You may be thinking, "I can't possibly go straight from reactive to creative!" And you're right—ordinarily, this shift seems impossible on the vibrational scale, especially depending on how you interpret the word "creative."

But here's the good news: I'm not asking you to compose a symphony, paint a three-metre masterpiece, or prepare a culinary feast. For this exercise, I'm asking you to **create space**. Create softness. Create allowing. Create a place within your body for your energy to come home.

The Practice:

1. Feel into your reactivity. Notice where it sits in your body. Now take three calming breaths. This may feel difficult if you want the outburst, if you're desperate to dispel that energy. Take the three breaths anyway—we'll deal with the energy in just a moment.

2. Create a space within your body for your energy to return. Bring it back to you in whatever way feels right. You might focus on your heart or a place deep in your belly. You might visualize your energy returning like a retractable vacuum cleaner cord. You might imagine bringing your light back to shine inward into your own body and away from whatever triggered the reaction. Consciously create softness and allowing.

3. Take as long as you need. You'll notice almost instantly: less restriction, less tightness in your body. Your energy is home.

4. Release or reschedule. If the timing is appropriate, you can deal with the energy of the trigger here and now. Do a round of tapping while acknowledging the anger (or whatever emotion was triggered), or simply acknowledge the reactivity. Alternatively, use your journal to write about it and let it go. If the timing isn't appropriate, set yourself a reminder to journal or tap later in the day.

Note: The purpose of this exercise is to soften into possibility. When we remain in a heightened or reactive state, we inadvertently create stress or illness in our bodies and cut ourselves off from the solutions and peace that are available to us. We are never doing these exercises to shut off or squash down our anger or emotions, but rather redirect that energy to allow something better.

Releasing Self-Doubt Tapping meditation

Before you begin; refer to the EFT tapping information on *Page 165* of this book for an explanation of tapping points and more information about how the Emotional Freedom Technique works. Try the detailed tapping example for *Releasing Shame and Guilt*.

Find a quiet place where you will be undisturbed for about 15 minutes.

Say out loud "I can't do anything right". Rate – 0-10.

Karate Chop - repeat 3 times while tapping - choose one, rotate all three, or choose your own specific statement.

- "Even though I doubt myself constantly, I choose to trust in my own worth".
- "Even though self-doubt has held me back, I'm ready to believe in myself".

- "Even though I question everything I do, I choose confidence over doubt".

Round 1: Acknowledging

- EB - I doubt myself so much
- SE - I question every decision I make
- UE - I feel this self-doubt weighing me down
- UN - Doubting my abilities and my worth
- CH - Feeling like I'm not good enough
- CB - Questioning if I can do anything right
- UA - This self-doubt that feels so real
- CR - All this doubt I've been carrying

Take a deep breath and release.
Round 2: Leaning Toward Letting Go

- KC – Even though this self-doubt has been so strong, I am ready to release it.
- EB - What if this doubt isn't the truth?
- SE - I can acknowledge doubt without believing it
- UE - This self-doubt has kept me small
- UN - I'm ready to release what's holding me back
- CH - Self-doubt was my survival, but I'm safe now
- CB - I can honour my doubt and let it go
- UA - I'm allowed to trust myself
- CR - I can be capable without doubting myself

Take a deep breath and release.

Round 3: Empowerment

- KC – Even though I doubted myself, I now release this self-doubt that no longer serves me.
- EB - I choose trust over doubt
- SE - I transform doubt into confidence
- UE - My power comes from believing in myself
- UN - I am capable, worthy, and enough
- CH - I am at peace with who I am
- CB - I reclaim my confidence from doubt
- UA - I am free from self-doubt
- CR - I am capable and I trust myself

Take a deep breath and release. Notice how you feel now.
Say out loud "I doubt myself". Rate 0-10. Repeat the tapping if you are still above a 2-3.

Setting Boundaries Practices

Boundaries feel scary when you've lived with DV. You've been punished for saying no, for having needs, for taking up space. You were never allowed to have boundaries. This exercise helps you practice boundary-setting in safe, small ways so you can rebuild that muscle. This exercise will continue over a period of time, it is not a sit down and do once exercise. Boundaries will feel uncomfortable at first. That's normal. Your body has been trained to fear consequences. Remind yourself:

- Discomfort doesn't mean danger
- Their disappointment /reaction is not your business
- You are allowed to have needs

1: Become aware of saying "Yes" when you mean "No".

For the next few days, simply notice when you say yes but feel no inside. Don't change anything yet—just observe. Journal:

- What was the request?
- What did you feel in your body? (tightness, heaviness, anxiety?)
- What were you afraid would happen if you said no?

2: Set a boundary with a safe person

Choose ONE small boundary to practice with someone safe—a trusted friend, therapist, or supportive family member. Start small:

- "I need to get off the phone now".
- "I'd prefer to meet for coffee instead of dinner".
- "I'm not up for visitors today".

Notice: The world doesn't end. They likely respond with understanding. Journal what happened.

3: Set a boundary for yourself

Self-care IS boundary-setting. Practice saying no to your own harsh inner voice:

- When you catch yourself saying "I should..." ask "Do I actually want to?"
- Set one non-negotiable self-care boundary this week (e.g., "I will not skip meals," "I will take 10 minutes alone each day," "I will not apologize for resting".)

Use your journal to record how you felt and what happened.

4 . Practice feeling into the energy of requests from others

When something comes up, pause before answering. A pause is not a bad thing, and most pauses will go unnoticed. You don't need to immediately fill a space with an answer. Take a deep belly breath and feel into how the request feels.

Does it feel jarring? Does a feeling or "lump" come up in your throat or stomach? Does it feel safe or ok?

When you are ready to answer, acknowledge their request and say your boundary. It's ok, you got this!!

"I understand [acknowledge their request], but it's a no from me, I need [your boundary]".

Examples:

- "I understand you'd like help with that, but it's a no from me today as I need to prioritize my own tasks today".
- "I appreciate the invitation, thanks for asking, and it's a no this time as I need some quiet time this weekend".

5. Journal Reflection Questions:

Use your journal to reflect on your progress with setting boundaries.

- What happened when you set your boundary?
- How did your body feel before, during, and after?
- What did you learn about yourself?
- What's one boundary you'd like to practice next?

Be easy on yourself! Every so often I still have a moment where boundary setting feels scary. In these moments I use the *Quick version of The A+ instant reset* method. From this space I acknowledge the "scary boundary", breathe and then ask. This is surprisingly quick and when you practice a lot, it becomes your go to. If I get a feeling of "No", I say "No". If I get a feeling of either way is fine, I choose what feels best in the moment from a really good energetic space.

Quick version of The A+ instant reset.

A – Acknowledge the feelings. I am feeling _____ in my body.

A – Air – your reminder to breathe. In for five, out for eight, three times.

A – Allow something different using Ask or Affirm – What's the best that can happen? I am moving through this experience.

THE END?

Just a just cos note... Tonight is the 2nd night in a row (and only the third night since I have lived here) that I have taken a shower after dark!!!! Winning!!! (By candle light so I don't have to try and hear through the exhaust fan, and with the dogs inside... 3 in 8 n 1/2 months... I was always too worried in case someone was outside...

This was an entry from my journal from years ago. I was living in such fear after leaving the DV environment that I was only showering during daylight hours, because while showering I felt so vulnerable and defenceless. Nude, wet, exposed and unable to see or hear if someone approached the house. Some days, the fear was so overwhelming I wouldn't shower at all. Finally feeling safe enough to shower at night was a milestone I hadn't even recognized at the time. Looking back at that progress, I hadn't realized how deep I had been in despair and how far I had come from it. I recall standing glass jars behind the doors with a coin balanced on the rim, so if the door opened, it would hit the jar, the coin would drop into the glass and alert me of an intruder. I was truly living in survival mode, every action and every thought laced with the undertone of how I could stay safe.

Today I have an ever-growing tool caddy of information and practices that remind me of who I am when life encourages me to grow. I feel a sense of safety and contentment that I had never had in life—a sense of "I got this".

Something I learned through this whole DV experience and out the other side, was that I didn't have to become someone. I didn't have to aim high or set big goals. I didn't need to be the next big name in personal development. I didn't need to own a five-million-dollar home to prove to anyone that I made it. I just needed to be me—Divine, Intelligent, Vibrant and Authentic. And I realized there is no "there"—no finishing line to cross, no moment when I'd finally "arrive." The end happens when we leave the earth (and even that is a new beginning). Life is the journey itself.

I feel safe now. I am still studying and learning, but there is a peace and comfort to my life. I have plans, goals and dreams and none of them seem impossible. I dare to dream; I dare to share the dreams with others. Some of them I am still not sure how to achieve, but there is a quiet knowing in me that they will become my reality. And some of them have already come into being as I quietly worked towards shifting my vibration and becoming aligned with what I wanted in life.

My healing wasn't dramatic, sudden or instantaneous. I've never had a breakthrough moment, no big "ah ha!", no miraculous life changes for the better—though I desperately wanted one because I was so desperate for the proof that I was changing and becoming successful. So desperate to have a life I enjoyed and at the time, I wanted it NOW. I wanted the big bang reward for all my hard efforts! I did get the rewards, but I experienced small shifts that turned my life around. I had to learn to notice those subtle but powerful changes instead.

Some women will experience sudden breakthroughs, the life-changing penny drop, big wins, the fist pumps, high fives and miracles. Others will break through with quiet determination. But I know for sure, either way—loud and miraculous, or quietly stepping—is perfect and beautiful and should be embraced. Both paths lead to peace, strength and personal empowerment, so don't hold onto any expectations and continue the journey in whatever way feels best for you.

During this life with no endings, we embrace change, go with the flow, roll with the waves, be the observer of the seasons and all the beauty they bring to our lives. Each experience paves the way for the next. Learn to love the challenges, stay steady and calm in the face of perceived adversity and look at life with new perspectives as we step out of old ways of being.

Share what you have learned. Share your experience and your knowledge with those who ask, or those who seek it. Once I learned something, I assumed everyone knew it and I was reluctant to share, but this isn't the case. We each discover different wisdom at different times. You might read an entire book and find that only one or two insights truly land for you—those are your gems. What seems obvious to you now might be exactly the gem someone else needs to hear.

So, with peace in my heart, I wish you a journey filled with curiosity, joy and growth. A new path to walk that you take

THE END?

step by step in your being of the DIVA that you are, with complete awareness of yourself, the world and the way you perceive it. Leave behind the old and step boldly into the new, knowing there is love and support here for you always—you only need ask.

You are and I am Divine, Intelligent, Vibrant and Authentic

With blessings from the DIVA who's been there... ;-)

THE CYCLE OF VIOLENCE

Domestic violence follows a predictable pattern known as the cycle of violence. This cycle consists of four distinct phases that repeat over time: the Honeymoon phase, the Tension-Building phase, the Aggression phase, and the Justification phase. Understanding this cycle is crucial because it explains why leaving an abusive relationship is so difficult—each phase plays a specific role in keeping victims trapped. The honeymoon phase offers hope and reinforces the emotional bond, while the other phases create fear, confusion, and self-doubt. Over time, the cycle typically speeds up and the violence intensifies, but the pattern remains the same. Recognizing these phases can help you understand that the abuse is not your fault and that the cycle itself is the problem.

1. Honeymoon Phase

The honeymoon phase mirrors the beginning of the relationship—when gifts, attention, and declarations of love felt genuine and exciting. In a healthy relationship, these gestures are simply part of building connection. But in an abusive relationship, these same behaviours become a tool within the cycle of violence.

After an abusive incident, the perpetrator returns to those early relationship behaviours: the apologies, the promises, the affection that made you fall in love in the first place. This is why the honeymoon phase is so powerful—it taps into the memory of who you believed your partner to be and creates hope that the "real" person is back. It's what keeps you believing that change is possible, and that the relationship can return to how it felt in the beginning.

Perpetrator's Behaviour: The perpetrator becomes apologetic, affectionate, and promises change. They may shower the victim with gifts, attention, and declarations of love. They appear genuinely remorseful, may cry, and promise "it will never happen again". They might attend counselling, stop drinking, or make other visible efforts to demonstrate their commitment to change. The perpetrator works hard to convince the victim that they've seen the error of their ways.

Victim's Feelings: The victim feels hopeful, relieved, and wants to believe the relationship can work. She sees glimpses of the person she fell in love with and feels validated that her love and patience are finally paying off. There's often a sense of joy mixed with cautious optimism. She may feel grateful for the peace and attention, sometimes even feeling responsible for "helping" her partner become better. This phase reinforces her emotional investment in the relationship.

2. Tension-Building Phase

Perpetrator's Behaviour: The perpetrator becomes increasingly irritable, critical, and unpredictable. Small issues trigger disproportionate anger. They may use passive-aggressive tactics, give the silent treatment, or make snide comments. Communication becomes difficult as the perpetrator finds fault with everything. There's a palpable sense of walking on eggshells. The perpetrator may increase controlling behaviours, monitoring the victim's activities, or isolating her from support systems.

Victim's Feelings: The victim feels anxious, hypervigilant, and constantly on edge. She tries desperately to keep the peace, anticipating the perpetrator's needs and adjusting her behaviour to avoid triggering an explosion. She feels confusion about what she's doing wrong and may blame herself for the mounting tension. There's an exhausting sense of trying to be "perfect" while knowing, deep down, that an explosion is inevitable. She may feel isolated and afraid to reach out for help.

3. Aggression/Explosion Phase

Perpetrator's Behaviour: The perpetrator releases the built-up tension through verbal, emotional, physical, sexual, or financial abuse. This can include screaming, name-calling, physical violence, threats, destruction of property, or sexual coercion. The abuse is often unpredictable in its severity and may escalate over time. The perpetrator loses control (or appears to) and directs their rage at the victim. They may blame the victim for "causing" their reaction.

Victim's Feelings: The victim experiences fear, shock, and trauma. Even if she anticipated the explosion, the reality is terrifying. She may dissociate or go into survival mode, focusing only on protecting herself (and/or her children if she has them). Afterward, she feels shaken, hurt, and deeply wounded—both physically and emotionally. There's often disbelief that someone who claims to love her could treat her this way. She may feel trapped, ashamed, and unsure of where to turn.

4. Justification/Rationalization Phase

Perpetrator's Behaviour: The perpetrator minimizes the abuse, denies its severity, or shifts blame entirely onto the victim. They might say things like "you made me do it", "it wasn't that bad", or "you're too sensitive". The perpetrator may claim they don't remember the incident or was provoked beyond reason. They avoid taking genuine responsibility and instead focus on justifying their actions or making the victim doubt her own experience of what happened.

Victim's Feelings: The victim experiences confusion and self-doubt. The perpetrator's explanations can make her question her own perception of reality (gaslighting). She may start to believe she is partly or fully responsible for the abuse. There's often a desperate need to make sense of what happened, which can lead her to accept the perpetrator's version of events. She may feel guilty, ashamed, or even protective of the perpetrator. This phase often blurs into the beginning of the honeymoon phase, as the victim becomes worn down and more vulnerable to reconciliation.

The cycle repeats with increasing frequency and severity over time, making it progressively harder for victims to break free. Understanding these phases can help survivors recognize the pattern and realize the abuse is not their fault.

ADDITIONAL INFORMATION

Integration and sustainability

Remember that vibrational healing is not about maintaining a constantly high frequency—that's neither realistic nor necessary. It's about developing the awareness and tools to recognize when your vibration has been affected by external influences and having practical ways to return to your authentic energetic state.

The goal is not perfection but rather conscious participation in your own energetic well-being. Each time you choose to shift your vibration back toward love and self-worth, you're not only healing yourself but contributing to the healing of the collective consciousness around domestic violence and all forms of harm.

As you practice these techniques, you'll likely notice that your tolerance for lower vibrational situations naturally decreases. This is a sign of healing—as you raise your vibration, you naturally attract and create experiences that match your new energetic state, making it easier to maintain healthy boundaries and relationships.

Daily Integration: Creating Your New Reality

Think of your healing journey like knitting or sewing a beautiful, warm blanket. You wouldn't sit down and try to knit an entire blanket in one exhausting marathon session—that would leave you overwhelmed, with sore hands, and likely abandoning the project altogether. This mirrors my own experience in writing this book! It seemed like such an impossible task at first, but I sat down and did a little each day. Some days I wrote more than other days—it became my blanket, woven thread by thread. The same has been true of my healing journey itself; showing up consistently, even in small ways, created transformation that trying to do it all at once never could. When you pick up your needles each day and knit a few rows, over time, something magnificent emerges. Each stitch matters. Each row adds to the whole. Some days you might knit more rows, other days just a few, but the consistency—not the intensity—is what creates the finished blanket that will comfort you for years to come.

Your healing practices work exactly the same way. The meditation you do for five minutes while your morning coffee brews, the EFT tapping sequence you complete in your car before walking into work, the moment you pause to take three conscious breaths before responding to a stressful text—these are your daily stitches. Individually, they might seem small. Together, over time, they weave a new reality.

Why Integration Matters

Integration is how you build a bridge between the woman you're becoming and the life you're living right now. It's how temporary insights become permanent shifts. It's how practices become second nature, and how your new authentic self gets woven into the fabric of your daily existence.

Without integration, healing remains theoretical, and you end up on a path of always trying to heal, always trying to fix. With integration, healing becomes your living reality, you heal.

Practice: Creating Your Sustainability Blueprint

This exercise will help you design a realistic, sustainable approach to maintaining your vibrational healing practices. You'll need your journal and about 20 minutes of uninterrupted time—and yes, you have 20 minutes. It's less time than we often spend procrastinating about doing the thing we need to do! (and less time than most spend scrolling on social media). Choose you.

Step 1: Identify Your "Morning Coffee Moments"

These are the small pockets of time that already exist in your day—transition moments that you can attach a practice to without adding anything extra to your schedule.

Write down 5-7 moments in your typical day:

- The time it takes your coffee to brew
- While you're in the shower
- During your commute (if you're not driving)

- In the bathroom (yes, really—privacy matters!)
- While waiting for your computer to start up
- Before you check your phone in the morning
- The last five minutes before sleep

Step 2: Match Practices to Moments

Now, beside each moment, write one simple practice that would fit naturally:

- *Coffee brewing:* 3-minute morning gratitude meditation
- *In the shower:* Speaking your "I am" affirmations aloud
- *Commute:* EFT tapping for releasing anxiety
- *Computer starting:* Three conscious breaths + intention setting
- *Before phone check:* Quick body scan—where am I holding tension?
- *Before sleep:* Forgiveness meditation or visualization

The key is matching the practice to the energy of the moment. Don't try to do an energizing practice right before sleep or a calming one when you need to gear up for the day.

Step 3: Start With Three Stitches

From your list, circle only THREE practices to begin with. Yes, just three. This is crucial. You're building a habit of consistency, not trying to overhaul your entire life overnight.

Choose:

- One morning practice
- One midday practice
- One evening practice

Commit to these three for the next 21 days. Mark them in your calendar. Set gentle reminders on your phone if helpful.

Now, I know what might be happening in this moment. You might be reading "commit to these for 21 days" and feeling that familiar weight in your chest. I understand, I felt it too! Twenty-one days to this, 30 days to that. It felt like too much, too big a task. I was sure I would fail before I even started, so why bother?

Here's what I learned: don't actually commit to 21 days. Don't commit to 30 days. Every day, just commit to tomorrow.

Tonight, before you sleep, journal your "intention for tomorrow" (you'll find this prompt in *My Diva Journal*, the companion to this book). That's it. Just one more day. Then tomorrow night, you do it again. One more day.

You're not climbing a mountain in one exhausting push—you're taking one step, and then another, and then another. Before you know it, without the pressure of a finish line looming over you, you've done 21 days. Maybe even 30. But that's not because you white-knuckled your way through a commitment that felt impossible. It's because you showed up for yourself, one gentle day at a time.

Mark your three practices somewhere visible if it helps. Set gentle reminders on your phone. But most importantly, release the grip of "I must do this for X days or I've failed". You haven't failed if you miss a day. You simply begin again tomorrow.

Step 4: Track Your Weaving

Create a simple tracking system—it can be as basic as three checkboxes in your journal each day or a note in your phone. But here's the important part: you're not tracking perfection, you're tracking awareness.

Each day, note:

- Did I do the practice?
- How did I feel after? (one word is enough)
- What did I notice about my vibration today?

After 21 days, you'll have a tapestry of data about what works for your unique life and rhythm.

Step 5: The Sustainability Check-In

Every Sunday (or whatever day works for you), spend five minutes asking yourself:

- Which practices felt sustainable this week?
- Which felt like a struggle?
- Where did I notice the biggest shift in my energy?
- What needs to be adjusted for next week?

This isn't about judging yourself—it's about becoming a compassionate observer of your own patterns. Maybe you discover that evening meditation doesn't work because you're too tired, but a morning practice lights you up. Maybe you realize that EFT tapping in your car before entering your workplace creates a protective buffer that changes your entire day. This information is gold.

The Accumulation Principle

Here's what makes this approach so powerful: small, consistent practices accumulate in ways that dramatic but sporadic efforts never do.

If you meditate for five minutes every single day for a month, you've given yourself 150 minutes (2.5 hours) of meditation practice. That's substantial. But more importantly, you've sent your nervous system the message 30 times that you're worthy of this pause, this care, this returning to centre. You've created 30 opportunities to notice your patterns, witness your thoughts, and choose differently. You've woven 30 rows into your blanket.

Compare this to meditating for an hour once, feeling inspired, and then forgetting about it for weeks. The one-hour session might feel more impressive, but it doesn't create the neural pathways, the habit, or the sustainable shift that daily practice does.

Your healing isn't a sprint to a finish line—it's a gentle, persistent walking toward wholeness. Each step counts. Each practice matters. Each moment you choose yourself is a thread in the tapestry of your new life.

When You Drop the Needles

Because you will. There will be days, maybe even weeks, when life gets overwhelming, and your practices fall away. Your child gets sick. You change jobs. The holidays arrive. You're triggered by an interaction and find yourself in old patterns.

This is not failure. This is being human.

The difference between someone who heals and someone who stays stuck isn't that the healer never falls—it's that she picks up her needles again. Without self-judgment. Without shame. Without the story that she's "blown it" or "back at square one".

You simply notice: "Oh, I haven't meditated in a week. I can feel the difference in my energy", I certainly felt that difference! "I'm going to do a 3-minute breathing practice right now". And you do. That's it. That's the practice. The returning is as important as the practice itself.

Signs Your Practices Are Becoming Integrated

Over time, you'll notice these markers of true integration:

- You automatically take a conscious breath before responding to something triggering
- Your body reminds you when you haven't done your practice—you feel the difference
- The practices start to feel less like something you "should" do and more like coming home to yourself
- You notice you're handling situations that would have previously destabilized you with more ease

- Other people comment on a change in your energy (though you're not doing this for them)
- You find yourself naturally teaching these tools to others who are struggling
- The gap between being thrown off centre and returning to your authentic state gets shorter

These are the signs that your blanket is taking shape. That the healing is no longer something you're doing—it's becoming who you are.

Remember: You're not trying to become someone new. You're carefully, lovingly, persistently uncovering the vibrant, authentic, divine, intelligent woman who was always there beneath the trauma. Each practice is a stitch. Each day is a row. Each choice to return to yourself is an act of revolutionary self-love.

Keep weaving, beautiful one. The warmth you're creating will sustain you through every season ahead.

Working with triggers and setbacks

Let's be clear about something important: triggers and setbacks are not signs that you're failing at healing. They're not evidence that you're broken or that nothing is working. They're simply part of being human, and especially part of healing from trauma. Your nervous system learned to protect you in certain ways, and sometimes those old protective patterns get activated—even when you're doing everything "right".

The difference now is that you have tools. You have awareness. And most importantly, you have compassion for yourself when these moments arise. The goal isn't to never be triggered—it's to recognize when you are, have ways to support yourself through it, and return to your centre with a little more ease each time.

Recognizing Your Early Warning Signs

Your body often knows you're being triggered before your mind catches up. Learning to recognize your unique early warning signs can help you intervene earlier, before you're fully activated. Common signals include:

- A sudden tightness in your chest or throat
- Your breath becoming shallow or held
- Tension in your jaw, shoulders, or stomach
- A feeling of spaciness or disconnection
- An urge to flee, fight, or freeze
- Your mind racing or going blank
- Heat rising in your body or sudden coldness
- A sick feeling in your body

My unique early warning sign was a feeling I could only describe as my head becoming heavy—like it was wrapped in a wet towel with eye holes cut out. This was followed by a nauseous feeling in my gut and weakness flowing through my body. It was deeply uncomfortable.

Take a moment now to think about your personal pattern. What does your body do when you're starting to feel triggered? Knowing this is like having an early warning system that gives you a chance to use your tools before you're overwhelmed.

Your Tool Caddy for Triggered Moments

When you notice you're being triggered—whether through those early warning signs or because you're already activated—here are your go-to tools:

The Pause Protocol (use this first when possible): When triggered, pause and place your hand on your heart. Ask, "What past part of me is being activated right now?". Send love to that part without trying to fix or change anything. This prevents you from getting stuck in reactive patterns. Alternatively, just pause, feel into the trigger or discomfort, take a breath and breathe love into it. Use a gentle affirmation, "I'm ok right now", "Body, we are ok".

Tapping on Triggers (especially helpful for intense activation): To feel instant relief after being triggered, simply tap on the karate chop point and acknowledge the feeling or the trigger. Use your breath to calm your body and nervous system as you tap. Tap gently on each of the points in order as you continue acknowledging the trigger. You don't need a script for this—just tap. You can gently replay any memory, let your body know you are safe, and continue to tap in this way for a couple of rounds or until the feeling subsides.

Additional tools in this book that support you through triggers and setbacks: Simple Breathing Technique (Part 1), Three Way Alignment Meditation (Part 2), and The A+ Instant Reset (Part 3).

Reframing Setbacks (for the self-judgment that often follows): When you notice your vibration dropping, instead of judging yourself, say, "I'm having a human experience, and that's okay. This is information, not a reflection of my worth". This keeps you from spiralling into shame or self-judgment, which only lowers your vibration further.

The Completion Technique (after a difficult interaction or before sleep): When you've been in a difficult situation or conversation, take a moment to energetically complete it. Take three deep breaths and say, "I release any energy that isn't mine. I call back any of my energy that scattered. I am whole and complete". You can also complete difficult moments before you sleep by doing a recapitulation of everything that occurred during the day. This allows you to release the day's energy—good or bad—and go to sleep clear.

After the Storm: Being Gentle with Yourself

Here's what often happens after we've been triggered: we use our tools, we start to feel better, and then we beat ourselves up for having been triggered in the first place. "Why did I react that way? I should be past this by now. I thought I was healed".

Please hear this: being triggered doesn't erase your progress. It doesn't mean you're back at the beginning. Your nervous system encountered something that reminded it of past danger, and it responded the way it was trained to respond. That's all. It's that simple. The fact that you noticed that you used tools to support yourself, that you're reading this right now, that's the healing.

Some days you'll catch the trigger early and shift quickly. Other days you might not remember your tools until hours later, or even the next day. Both of these are okay. There's no perfect way to do this. What matters is that you keep returning to yourself with kindness.

If you find yourself triggered and completely forget about all your tools in the moment, that's information too. It tells you that particular trigger runs deep, or that you might need more support around it. It doesn't mean you've failed. Tomorrow, or the next time, you might remember one tool. And the time after that, you might remember even sooner. This is how healing actually works—not in a straight line, but in a gentle spiral that gradually brings you home to yourself.

Be patient with your nervous system. It's learning a new language. It's learning that it's safe to feel, safe to stay present, safe to respond rather than react. That learning takes time, repetition, and above all, compassion.

The Heart, Brain, Gut Connection

Your body has three intelligence centres that are constantly communicating: your brain, your heart, and your gut. What I didn't realize is that my heart contains around 40,000 specialized neurons—a complex neural network that allows it to sense, learn, and remember independently of the brain in my head. Similarly, the gut houses around 100 million neurons in what scientists call the enteric nervous system, often referred to as your "second brain." Brain cells are present in the brain, heart and gut.

When you're stressed or anxious, these three centres fall out of sync—they're sending conflicting signals to each other, creating a state of incoherence that you experience as anxiety, scattered thinking, or physical tension. Meditation works by bringing all three intelligence centres into rhythmic alignment.

The slow, intentional breathing pattern (especially the extended exhale) activates your vagus nerve—the body's main communication highway that runs from your brainstem down through your neck and branches throughout your torso, connecting your brain with your heart, gut, and other vital organs. This signals your nervous system to shift from "fight or flight" into "rest and digest" mode. By placing attention on your heart while breathing rhythmically, you're creating a harmonious pattern that your heart communicates to your brain and throughout your body via electromagnetic signals and neural pathways.

When these three centres align, you experience a cascade of benefits: clearer thinking, emotional balance, reduced stress hormones, and access to your deeper intuition. This state of alignment allows your body's natural wisdom to emerge—the kind of knowing that doesn't come from thinking harder, but from listening deeper.

Why This Matters for Trauma Recovery

For someone recovering from domestic violence, heart, brain, gut alignment exercises can be particularly powerful for:

1. *Emotional Regulation*: The ability to alter one's emotional responses is central to overall well-being and to effectively meeting the demands of life. Heart coherence helps you regain control over your emotional responses.
2. *Nervous System Reset*: Trauma dysregulates your nervous system. Heart coherence exercises help restore balance between your sympathetic (fight-or-flight) and parasympathetic (rest-and-digest) nervous systems.
3. *Body-Mind Integration*: The heart-brain connection means that when you create coherence in your heart, you're directly influencing your mental and emotional state from the body up, rather than trying to think your way out of trauma responses.
4. *Cellular Communication*: The "heart brain" communicates within the body neurologically, hormonally, and energetically, from second to second with the trillions of cells in your body. This means coherence affects your entire system.

EMOTIONAL FREEDOM TECHNIQUE

What is EFT?

EFT (Emotional Freedom Techniques) is a therapeutic tool that combines elements of cognitive therapy with acupressure. It involves tapping with your fingertips on specific meridian points on the body while focusing on a particular issue or emotion.

How Does It Work?

The theory behind EFT is that negative emotions are caused by disruptions in the body's energy system. By tapping on meridian endpoints (used in acupuncture) while acknowledging the problem, you:

- Send calming signals to the amygdala (the brain's alarm system)
- Reduce the stress response associated with the emotional issue

- Rewire the brain's reaction to triggers and memories

The Basic Process:

1. **Identify the issue** - What emotion or problem you're addressing (e.g., shame, fear, anxiety)
2. **Rate the intensity** - On a scale of 0-10, how intense is the feeling or how true does it feel?
3. **The Setup Statement** - Tap on the "karate chop" point while saying: "Even though I feel/have (this problem), I deeply and completely accept myself" (acknowledging).
4. **The Tapping Sequence** - Tap on each meridian point (about 5-7 taps each) while repeating reminder phrases about your topic.
5. **Re-rate the intensity** - Check if the emotional charge has decreased.

Why It's Effective for Trauma

EFT helps process difficult emotions without re-traumatizing because you're acknowledging the issue while simultaneously calming your nervous system through the tapping. It's particularly useful for shame, anxiety, and limiting beliefs—all common after DV.

Introduction to EFT Tapping

EFT (Emotional Freedom Techniques) is a powerful tool that combines gentle tapping on specific meridian points with focused intention to release emotional blocks and rewire your nervous system's response to challenging feelings and memories.

The Tapping Points (in sequence)

1. Karate Chop (KC) - Side of the hand (the fleshy part under the side of the little finger you'd use for a karate chop)
2. Eyebrow (EB) - Beginning of the eyebrow, just above the bridge of the nose
3. Side of Eye (SE) - On the bone at the outer corner of the eye
4. Under Eye (UE) - On the bone directly under the eye
5. Under Nose (UN) - Between the bottom of the nose and upper lip
6. Chin (CH) - In the crease between your lower lip and chin
7. Collarbone (CB) - Just below the collarbone, about 5cm from centre
8. Under Arm (UA) - About 10cm below the armpit
9. Crown (CR) - Top of your head

How to Tap:

- Use 2-3 fingers
- Tap firmly but gently, about 5-7 times on each point
- You can tap on either side of the body, or both sides simultaneously
- Breathe naturally throughout

The Process:

1. Identify the issue and rate its intensity (0-10)
2. Create a setup statement: "Even though [problem], I deeply and completely accept myself"
3. Tap the Karate Chop point while saying the setup statement 3 times
4. Tap through all the other points while saying reminder phrases
5. Take a deep breath and re-rate the intensity
6. Repeat rounds as needed

Tapping Scripts
Notes on Using These Scripts

Personalize Them: Feel free to change words or phrases to match your specific situation. The more personal and specific you make them, the more powerful they'll be.

Repeat as Needed: If a particular issue still feels charged, Keep tapping until the intensity drops to a 2 or below. You don't have to do it all on the same day. Use your journal to write a note and choose another time to tap.

Daily Practice: The Daily Empowerment Practice can be used every morning to start your day aligned with your authentic power.

Trust the Process: EFT works even if you don't fully believe the positive statements at first. Your subconscious is listening, and change happens with repetition and practice.

Be Gentle: Some sessions may bring up emotions. This is normal and part of the healing process. Have tissues nearby and give yourself permission to feel whatever comes up.

Combine Techniques: These tapping scripts work beautifully alongside the other tools in this book - journaling, boundary-setting practices and mirror practices.

Remember: You are not broken. You are healing. Every time you tap, you're choosing yourself, your freedom, and your authentic power.

Releasing Shame and Guilt (Detailed Tapping Guide)

Take a moment to tune into any shame or guilt you're carrying. Notice where you feel it in your body. Rate the intensity of this feeling from 0-10 (with 10 being the most intense).

Say out loud – "I feel so ashamed and guilty". Rate this feeling on a scale of 0-10.

Setup Statement Options (Choose one, use all three or create your own):

"Even though I carry this deep shame about what happened to me, I choose to accept myself anyway".

"Even though I feel guilty for staying, for not seeing it sooner, for not protecting myself better, I deeply and completely accept myself".

"Even though shame tells me I'm fundamentally flawed, I acknowledge this feeling and choose self-compassion".

Tap on the Karate Chop Point (Say your set up statement 3 times while tapping): "Even though I carry this deep shame about what happened to me, I choose to accept myself anyway"

ROUND 1: Acknowledging
Tap through each point while saying the corresponding phrase.
Eyebrow: This shame and guilt that I am carrying
Side of Eye: Shame tells me I'm fundamentally flawed
Under Eye: This guilt I feel for staying
Under Nose: The shame of what happened
Chin: Guilt for not seeing it sooner
Collarbone: This heavy shame in my body
Under Arm: All this guilt I've been holding
Crown: This guilt and shame is so uncomfortable
Take a deep breath and release. Move to round 2.

ROUND 2: Leaning Toward Letting Go
Karate Chop : "Even though this shame has been protecting me in some way, I'm open to releasing it now".
Eyebrow: What if this shame doesn't define me?
Side of Eye: I'm beginning to see shame for what it is
Under Eye: Maybe I can let some of this guilt go
Under Nose: This shame was never mine to carry
Chin: I'm open to releasing this heavy burden
Collar bone: Choosing to be gentle with myself
Under Arm: I survived, and that matters
Crown: Opening to the possibility of release
Take a deep breath and release. Move onto round 3.

ROUND 3: Empowerment

Karate Chop: "I choose to release this shame and guilt and reclaim my worth"
Eyebrow: I am not what happened to me
Side of Eye: I choose self-compassion over shame
Under Eye: I release this guilt that was never mine
Under Nose: I am worthy, just as I am
Chin: I survived, and I'm still here
Collarbone: I choose to honour my journey
Under Arm: I am whole, not broken
Crown: I reclaim my voice and my worth

Take a deep breath and release. Notice how you feel now.

Say out loud, "I feel so ashamed and guilty". Rate this feeling on a scale of 0-10.

If it's still above a 2-3, you can do another round focusing on whatever aspect still feels charged.

Use the following tapping meditations in the same way as the detailed version, rating the intensity before and after your tapping.

Release Being a Victim

Say out loud "I am a victim" Rate – 0-10.

Karate Chop - repeat 3 times while tapping - choose one, rotate all three, or choose your own specific statement.

"Even though I was a victim of abuse, I choose to reclaim my power now".

"Even though I've been living in victim identity, I'm ready to transform".

"Even though being the victim felt safe, I'm ready to step into my strength".

Round 1: Acknowledging
EB - I am such a victim
SE - That part is real and undeniable
UE - I lived through something terrible
UN - I was hurt and harmed
CH - This victim identity kept me safe
CB - It helped people understand what I went through
UA - But it's become a prison of its own
CR – I'm afraid no one will believe me if I'm not the victim anymore

Take a deep breath and release.

Round 2: Leaning Toward Letting Go
KC – Even though I am a victim, I am open to releasing being a victim now
EB - What if I could honour what happened without staying stuck?
SE - I can acknowledge I was victimized without being a victim
UE - That was something that happened to me, not who I am
UN - I'm ready to release this identity
CH - I'm more than what was done to me
CB - I survived, and that makes me a survivor not a victim
UA - I can be strong and still honour my pain
CR - Letting go of the victim story

Take a deep breath and release.

Round 3: Empowerment
KC – What if I honour what happened and choose to move forward?
EB - I am not a victim, I am a survivor
SE - I choose to reclaim my power
UE - I define myself now, not my past
UN - I am strong, capable, and whole
CH - My story is one of resilience, not defeat
CB - I am the author of my life now
UA - I choose empowerment over victimhood
CR - I reclaim my strength

Take a deep breath and release. Notice how you feel now.
Say out loud, "I am a victim". Rate – 0-10. Repeat the tapping if you are still above a 2-3.

Releasing Anger
Say out loud "I am so angry". Rate – 0-10.
Karate Chop - repeat 3 times while tapping - choose one, rotate all three, or choose your own specific statement.

"Even though I have every right to be angry, I choose to release this rage for my own peace".

"Even though this anger has been burning inside me, I'm ready to let it go".

"Even though I'm furious about what happened, I choose freedom over fury".

Round 1: Acknowledging
EB - I am so angry I feel it in my body
SE - I have every right to be furious
UE - I feel intense anger at this injustice
UN - Furious that this happened
CH - Angry at myself for staying
CB - Rage at a world that didn't protect me
UA - This anger that feels justified
CR - All this rage I've been holding onto
Take a deep breath and release.

Round 2: Leaning Toward Letting Go
KC – Even though this anger has been so intense, I am ready to release it.
EB - What if holding this anger is hurting me most?
SE - I can be angry and still choose peace
UE - This rage has served its purpose
UN - I'm ready to release what's burning me
CH - Anger was my protection, but I'm safe now
CB - I can honour my anger and let it go
UA - I'm allowed to release it
CR - I can be strong without staying angry
Take a deep breath and release.

Round 3: Empowerment
KC – Even though I was so angry, I now release this anger that no longer serves me.
EB - I choose peace over rage
SE - I transform anger into strength

UE - My power comes from within, not from anger
UN- I am calm, centered, and strong
CH - I am at peace with myself
CB - I reclaim my energy from anger
UA - I am free from fury
CR - I am powerful and at peace

Take a deep breath and release. Notice how you feel now.
Say out loud "I am so angry". Rate 0-10. Repeat the tapping if you are still above a 2-3.

Releasing Anxiety and Fear
Say out loud "I am so scared and anxious". Rate – 0-10.
Karate Chop - repeat 3 times while tapping - choose one, rotate all three, or choose your own specific statement.

"Even though this anxiety and fear control so much of my life, I choose to feel safe now".

"Even though I'm always waiting for something to go badly, I choose peace".

"Even though fear keeps me hypervigilant, I'm safe enough to relax now".

Round 1: Acknowledging
EB - This constant anxiety, I can't do this anymore
SE - Fear running through my veins
UE - Always waiting for something bad to happen
UN – I am so afraid of_____
CH - Anxiety about the future
CB - Fear that I'm not safe, I'll never be safe!

UA - This nervous energy in my body makes me feel sick
CR - This anxiety keeps me awake
Take a deep breath and release.

Round 2: Leaning Toward Letting Go
KC – Even though I feel anxious, what if I could feel safe in this moment?
EB - My body learned to be afraid, it can learn to be calm
SE - Opening to the possibility of peace
UE - This anxiety has protected me
UN - My nervous system can learn to rest
CH - I'm allowed to feel calm
CB - Letting go of always waiting for danger or something bad to happen
UA - Opening to peace and ease
CR - Ready to release this fear
Take a deep breath and release.

Round 3: Empowerment
KC – Even though it's been so hard, I am willing to allow something better
EB - I choose peace over anxiety
SE - My body knows how to be calm
UE - I release fear and embrace safety
UN - I can trust myself to handle whatever comes
CH - I choose ease over hypervigilance
CB - I am safe, I am calm, I am at peace
UA - My nervous system is healing
CR - I release all fear

Take a deep breath and release. Notice how you feel now.

Say out loud "I am so scared and anxious". Rate – 0-10. Repeat the tapping if your number is still above 2-3.

Empowering the Self

Say out loud "I am so small and powerless". How true does this feel? Rate – 0-10.

Karate Chop - repeat 3 times while tapping - choose one, rotate all three, or choose your own specific statement.

"Even though I've felt powerless for so long, I choose to reclaim my strength".

"Even though I forgot how powerful I am, I'm remembering now".

"Even though I was taught to stay small, I choose to step into my power".

Round 1: Acknowledging
EB - I've felt so powerless
SE - Like I had no control over my life
UE - I was taught to stay small
UN - To not take up space
CH - To doubt my own strength
CB – I'm uncertain of what I'm capable of
UA - I've been diminished for so long
CR - Acknowledging where I am

Round 2: Leaning Toward Letting Go

KC - Even though I have felt small, I am learning I am more powerful than I know.

EB - I survived everything that tried to break me
SE - That took incredible strength
UE - I'm beginning to see my resilience
UN - I'm ready to stop playing small
CH - My strength has been here all along
CB - I'm allowed to take up space
UA - Ready to step into who I truly am
CR - Opening to my full potential

Round 3: Empowerment

KC - Even though I have struggled, I am open to something amazing

EB - I am powerful beyond measure
SE - I reclaim my strength and my voice
UE - I am capable of anything I set my mind to
UN - I am strong, resilient, and brave
CH - I honour the power within me
CB - I take up space unapologetically
UA - I am worthy of all good things
CR - My power comes from my authentic self

Say out loud "I am so small and powerless". How true does this feel now? Rate – 0-10.

Tapping into Divine

Say out loud "I have lost faith in the divine". How true does this feel? Rate – 0-10.

Karate Chop - repeat 3 times while tapping - choose one, rotate all three, or choose your own specific statement.

"Even though I've felt disconnected from something greater, I choose to reconnect now".

"Even though I've lost faith in the universe, I'm open to divine guidance".

"Even though I've felt alone in this journey, I'm opening to divine support".

Round 1: Acknowledging
EB - I've feel so disconnected, separated from something greater
SE - The trauma cut me off from my spiritual self
UE - I've felt alone in this universe
UN - I don't understand why this happened to me
CH - I feel abandoned by the universe
CB - I can't access divine wisdom
UA - Feeling like I'm doing this life thing alone
CR - Unable to trust in anyone, anything or myself

Round 2: Leaning Toward Letting Go
KC – Even though I have felt incredibly alone, I am open to the possibility of divine support.
EB - Maybe the universe has been guiding me all along
SE - Ready to reconnect with something greater
UE - I can trust in the universe again
UN - Allowing spiritual connection to return
CH - The divine has always been within me
CB - I'm ready to listen to divine guidance

UA - Opening my heart to universal love
CR - Ready to feel connected again

Round 3: Empowerment
KC – Even though divine connection felt impossible, I am allowing infinite possibilities.
EB - I am open to being supported by the universe
SE - I trust in divine guidance
UE - I am a spiritual being having a human experience
UN -- The divine flows through me
CH - I am never alone
CB - I trust in the unfolding of my journey
UA - I am divinely guided and protected
CR - I honour the divine within me

Say out loud "I have lost faith in the divine". How true does this feel now? Rate – 0-10.

Tapping into Intelligent

Say out loud "I'm just not smart and I make crappy decisions". How true does this feel?
Rate – 0-10.

Karate Chop - repeat 3 times while tapping - choose one, rotate all three, or choose your own specific statement.

"Even though I've doubted my intelligence and judgment, I choose to trust my wisdom now".

"Even though I was made to feel stupid, I reclaim my brilliant mind".

"Even though I've questioned my decisions, I trust my intelligence".

Round 1: Acknowledging
EB - I've doubted my intelligence
SE - Was told I was stupid, crazy, wrong
UE - Made to question my own judgment
UN - I was constantly criticized
CH - I can't trust my own mind
CB - Doubting every choice I make
UA - This feeling of not being smart enough
CR - Afraid to trust my own thinking

Round 2: Leaning Toward Letting Go
KC - What if my intelligence has been here all along?
EB - My mind is sharp and capable
SE - I'm ready to trust my judgment again
UE - I can trust my own thinking
UN - Letting go of others' voices in my head
CH - I'm allowed to trust myself and my decisions
CB - Ready to reclaim my intellectual power
UA - Opening to my natural intelligence
CR - I am wiser than I know

Round 3: Empowerment
KC – Even though I have had doubts about my intelligence, I am on the path to trusting myself.
EB - I am intelligent and capable
SE - I trust my mind and my judgment

UE - I make excellent decisions
UN - I trust my intellectual abilities
CH - My mind is powerful and clear
CB - I trust myself completely
UA - I am wise beyond measure
CR - I reclaim my intellectual power

Say out loud "I'm just not smart and I make crappy decisions". How true does this feel now?
Rate – 0-10.

Tapping into Vibrant
Say out loud "I feel drained, tired and depleted". How true does this feel in your body?
Rate – 0-10.
Karate Chop - repeat 3 times while tapping - choose one, rotate all three, or choose your own specific statement.

"Even though I've felt drained and depleted, I choose to reclaim my vibrancy".

"Even though my spark has dimmed, I'm ready to shine again".

"Even though I've been surviving instead of thriving, I choose vitality now".

Round 1: Acknowledging
EB - I've felt so drained
SE - My energy has been depleted
UE - Just surviving, not thriving
UN - I've been running on empty

CH - This exhaustion in my bones
CB - Life has felt heavy, grey and hard all the time
UA - I've lost my vibrancy and my joy
CR - I miss feeling alive

Round 2: Leaning Toward Letting Go
KC - What if I could feel alive again?
EB - I'm ready to reclaim my energy
SE – I am open to rediscovering vitality again
UE - I can feel vibrant and alive
UN - Letting go of constant exhaustion
CH - I give myself permission to feel good again
CB - Ready to thrive, not just survive
UA - Opening to seeing life's beauty
CR - I'm coming back to life

Round 3: Empowerment
KC – I am open to feeling vibrant
EB - I reclaim my energy and vitality
SE - I am alive, awake, and thriving
UE - Joy flows through me
UN - I am radiant and bright
CH - I choose vibrancy in every moment
CB - I allow myself to shine brightly in this world
UA - I am individual, beautiful and vibrant
CR - I reclaim my spark

Say out loud "I feel drained, tired and depleted". How true does this feel in your body now?

Rate – 0-10.

Tapping into Authentic

Say out loud "I have completely lost touch with who I really am. I don't know myself". How true does this feel in your body? Rate – 0-10.

Karate Chop - repeat 3 times while tapping - choose one, rotate all three, or choose your own specific statement.

"Even though I've been hiding behind personas, I choose to show up as my true self".

"Even though I've lost touch with who I really am, I'm ready to rediscover myself".

"Even though being authentic feels scary, I choose truth over performance".

Round 1: Acknowledging
EB - I've been hiding my true self
SE - Wearing masks to stay safe
UE - I've lost touch with who I really am
UN - Been performing my life instead of living it
CH - People-pleasing to survive
CB - Editing myself to fit in
UA - Afraid to show the real me
CR – I've been living behind a veil

Round 2: Leaning Toward Letting Go
KC - What if it's safe to be myself now?
EB - My authentic self has been waiting
SE - She's been here all along

UE - I'm ready to remove the masks
UN - Letting go of the need to perform
CH - My authentic voice deserves to be heard
CB - I'm allowed to be me
UA - My genuine self is emerging
CR - I'm safe enough to be real now

Round 3: Empowerment
KC – What if it is safe to be authentically, unapologetically myself?
EB - I honour my truth and speak my voice
SE - I show up as my whole, real self
UE - I am genuine and true
UN - I trust my authentic nature
CH - I live in alignment with my values
CB - My authenticity is my power
UA - I am real, raw, and beautiful
CR - I am safe

Say out loud "I have completely lost touch with who I really am. I don't know myself". How true does this feel in your body now? Rate – 0-10.

Daily Empowerment Practice

You may choose to do a rating on this one if you don't feel empowered. Otherwise, just enjoy this empowering practice!

Karate Chop - repeat 3 times while tapping - choose one, rotate all three, or choose your own specific statement.

"I choose to start this day connected to my power".

"I honour myself and my journey today".
"I am worthy of all good things coming to me today".

Round 1: Grounding in the Present
EB - I am here in this moment now
SE - I honour where I am today even if I feel a little off, it's all ok
UE - I release yesterday's struggles
UN - I don't need to think about tomorrow
CH - Right now, in this moment, I am safe
CB - In this moment, I breathe in peace
UA - I am centered and calm
CR - I am present here and now and I am ok

Round 2: Opening to Possibility
KC – What if I can be open to infinite positive possibilities?
EB - I'm open to what today brings
SE - I trust myself to handle whatever comes
UE - I'm worthy of good things happening
UN - Opening to joy, peace, and ease
CH - I allow life to support me
CB - I'm open to unexpected blessings
UA - I trust in the unfolding of this day
CR - I'm ready for, and deserving, positive experiences

Round 3: Empowerment
KC – What if I really am powerful and capable?
EB - I trust myself completely

SE - I am worthy of love, joy, and peace
UE - I am Divine, Intelligent, Vibrant, and Authentic
UN - I am aligned with my highest good
CH - I am exactly where I need to be right now
CB - I am enough, right now, as I am
UA - I choose empowerment in every moment
CR - I am a DIVA! Divine, intelligent, vibrant and authentic

ADDITIONAL TOOLS & PRACTICES

Image In

I always thought the word imagine really was just a misspelling of image in! so when I think of anything I am imagining, I am thinking of imaging it in to my life, imaging it into my reality or imaging it into becoming or being. (And yes, you may have noticed, I love this play with letters!) There is a lot on the internet and in self help books about visualisation and it works on the premise of first seeing it in the mind , creating it on an energetic level and then being in the space of allowing it to come into physical reality.

I created myself a sign made from wood and it says (on purpose) *"Imagein"* and it's a reminder to me to be most aware of what I am imaging in. If I am in a state of despair and fearing the worst, I am having pictures in my mind of just that. This is a dangerous place to be in! and those images definitely need an upgrade to something far better. If you see something you don't want to see, you look away. If there is something on television or the internet that you don't want to watch, you change the channel. I encourage you to do the same with the images in your mind. They are always there, choose a channel, choose images, choose to image in that which will serve your life.

This practice is a gentle reminder to change the channel and choose healthy images. When you find yourself deep in despair, fearful of the future, or replaying frightening images of the past, become aware of it. Your emotions will usually guide you to this awareness—you'll be feeling afraid, sad, lonely, desperate, or fearful.

Where focus goes, energy flows. The more attention you give to scenes that have already happened in your life, the more you are imaging them in, and the more of that same energy you create. Replaying those old stories keeps you stuck in the same energy.

1. Begin with reminding yourself "I am aware".
2. Acknowledge and see the unwanted images that you have been looking at.
3. See the unwanted image turning from colour to black and white and allow it to become smaller and smaller until it fades completely.
4. Bring in your new image – this can be a related or unrelated image. It might be something you want to happen instead, or you might change the subject completely to something that makes you feel happy.

5. When you have your new image, turn up the boldness, the sharpness and the colour. Have your image grow larger and larger until its so big and bright, that it completely surrounds you. Let it get bigger and brighter and bolder!
6. Practice this anytime you become aware of yourself imaging in something unwanted or replaying old stories.

Examples;

Going over and over in your head a scene from the past that was frightening. Allow it to fade and bring in the image of sitting at dinner with friends, laughing and feeling good.

Seeing your wallet empty and noticing things are "expensive". Allow it to fade and bring in the image of your wallet full of cash and see yourself noticing affordable prices on the price tags.

Predicting the worst in a future scenario where you are afraid of what might happen. Allow that to fade and image in the scene as though it had already happened and it worked out for the best.

Cord cutting meditation

There are many practitioners who can guide you through a cord cutting exercise, but this one is simple and effective in releasing your attachment on an energetic level.

What Are Energetic Cords?

When we're in relationships, especially intense or traumatic ones, we create energetic connections with others.

These invisible "cords" can continue to drain your energy and keep you emotionally tied to someone even after the relationship has ended. Cutting these cords doesn't mean erasing memories or denying what happened—it means reclaiming your energy and freeing yourself from ongoing emotional entanglement.

The Practice:

Find a quiet, comfortable space where you won't be disturbed. Sit or lie down in a relaxed position.

1. **Ground and Protect:** Close your eyes and take three deep breaths. Visualize roots growing from the base of your spine deep into the earth, anchoring and grounding you. Now imagine a sphere of bright, protective white or golden light surrounding your entire body. This light keeps you safe and supported.
2. **Scan for Cords:** Bring to mind the person you wish to release. Notice where in your body you feel the connection—it might be your heart, solar plexus, throat, or gut. You may sense or visualize a cord of energy connecting you to this person.
3. **Acknowledge the Connection:** Without judgment, acknowledge this cord and what it represents. You might say silently or aloud: "I acknowledge this connection and what it has taught me. I honour my journey, and I am ready to release what no longer serves me".
4. **Call In Support:** Invite in whatever higher power, spiritual guides, or loving energy feels right to you—whether that's the Universe, God, your Higher

Self, an Angel or simply the energy of unconditional love. Ask for support in this release.

5. **Cut the Cord:** Visualize yourself holding scissors, a sword of light, or simply using your hand to cut through the cord. You might see the cord dissolve, burn away, or simply fall away. As you cut it, say: "I release you with love. I reclaim my energy. I am free".

6. **Seal and Heal:** Once the cord is cut, visualize the place where it was attached to you being filled with healing light—golden, white, or whatever colour feels nurturing to you. This light seals and heals the space, making you whole again. Take the piece that is still connected to the other person and 'plug' it into the Universe or God and allow them to be connected to something higher.

7. **Reclaim Your Energy:** Imagine all the energy you've been giving to this person flowing back to you like a warm, healing stream. Feel yourself becoming fuller, more vibrant, more present in your own body.

8. **Gratitude and Closure:** Place your hand on your heart and take three deep breaths. Thank yourself for doing this healing work. When you're ready, gently open your eyes.

After the Meditation:

You may need to repeat this practice multiple times, especially if the relationship was long or particularly traumatic. This is normal—deep cords take time to fully release. You might also notice emotions surfacing after cord cutting. Allow yourself to feel and process them with compassion.

Remember: Cutting cords doesn't mean you hate the person or wish them harm. It simply means you're choosing to stop giving your precious life force energy to someone who is no longer (or never was) healthy for you. This is an act of self-love and reclamation.

Blessing ball meditation

This is a beautiful way of feeling energy, for real! Find a comfortable place to sit quietly where you will not be disturbed. Close your eyes and take three cleansing, calming breaths .

Now hold your hands in front of you like you are holding a small basketball, with your palms facing each other. With your eyes still closed, gently push and pull your hands towards and away from each other. Within a few moments you will feel a magnetic like feeling or a tingling or warm feeling in your hands. This is your energy ball, or blessing ball. On your next breath, breathe love and light into your body and breathe out something beautiful into your blessing ball.

You might like to add some love for yourself, a pet, or a friend. A blessing for whoever needs it today. Gratitude, peace or prosperity. Add some health and wellbeing, some laughter, joy or anything else you would like to have in your life. You can make your blessing ball just for yourself, for you and others, or for the planet, nature and humanity as a whole.

Sit with your blessing ball for as long as you feel comfortable. When you are ready, turn your hands towards yourself to send the blessing ball to your own body, or turn your hands outward and send the blessing to your recipient.

Affirmations

I know affirmations feel like they have been done, but it stands that they are incredibly powerful. The main idea though is that the affirmation needs to be believable. If you don't believe in your affirmation, it won't be as beneficial. If you are using an affirmation that doesn't resonate with you it takes so much longer to take effect as it involves repetition until the mind begins to believe in the possibility. Whereas an affirmation that is believable will have a much quicker effect as there isn't the added challenge of disbelief involved. Don't say I am strong if you are not feeling strong.

1. Make yourself a list of affirmations or use some of these.

I am whole and complete exactly as I am.

I am divinely guided and protected. I trust the wisdom within me.

My value exists independent of anyone's opinion, choice, or validation.

I am trusting my intuition. My inner knowing has never led me astray.

I am capable of learning, growing, and making wise decisions for myself.

I am receiving so much good in my life.

I am vibrant, present, and worthy of joy in this moment.

My energy is precious, and I choose carefully where I invest it.

I am allowed to take up space, to shine, and to live boldly.

I am beautiful and intelligent.
I am living in peace and harmony.
I am enough, exactly as I am.

Try them for size!

Feel into each of these affirmations. Choose one and feel how it fits. Does it feel light or heavy, real or unreal. If it feels light, it's a match! If it feels a little off, try tweaking it.

1. Repeat your affirmations daily as many times a day as you can out loud or in your head.
2. Use the voice recorder on your phone to record some of your favourite affirmations. Play them in the car, while you take a bath, while you are cooking dinner.

Rewriting the language

Healing of body and mind begins when we start to question our language habits and replacing them with more accurate, compassionate language. Practice awareness of what you are saying to yourself and others by simply stating, "I am aware".

Instead of "How could I be so stupid?", try "I made the best decisions I could with the information and emotional resources I had at the time".

Instead of "My perpetrator" try using their name, a nickname if using their name is too triggering or simply their initials. By doing this, you are disassociating them with being connected to you or "yours".

Instead of "I should have known better", try "I was dealing with someone who was deliberately deceptive and manipulative".

Instead of "I'm weak for staying", try "I showed incredible strength by surviving and eventually finding my way out".

This shift is transformational. When we change how we speak to ourselves, we change how we see ourselves, our environment, and ultimately, how we heal. When we change how we speak about others and to others, our environment changes.

Be aware of chastising yourself. – "Oh, idiot", "I wish I had never…", "I was so stupid, what was I thinking?".

1. Say each day, throughout the day "I am aware".
2. Pause before speaking and ask, "is what I am about to say kind, necessary and true?". If the answer is "no" to any of these, choose something else to say.
3. Ask friends and family to help keep you accountable with your words. If you start delving into "that story" again, ask them to gently redirect you or remind you to choose another narrative. Also be aware of anyone else "holding" you in that story, and gently redirect.

Cleansing Negative Energy Meditation

I distinctly remember an icky feeling throughout my whole body that felt almost physical. Like my body was lined on the inside with a filthy black sticky layer of tar. It felt constricting. There are a few similar meditations to this one, but this is my version and I did it more than once! Like hosing mud off a dirty car, I hosed away the ickyness and felt wonderfully cleansed afterwards.

The Practice:

Close your eyes and take three cleansing breaths. Breathe in for 5 seconds and out for 7-8 seconds, allowing your belly to expand on the in breath and deflate on the out breath.

Now imagine you step into an elevator with a large bin beside you. The elevator is going to take you up into the inside of your head. From this viewpoint, you'll be able to see inside your head and down into your body as though you were looking into a tall building.

The elevator goes up and up, then stops. The door opens and you're standing inside your head. The walls may look curved or square, and you may see a black sticky coating on them. If you don't have a sticky coating, look around for dust or rubbish.

Next, take a hose and wash away the coating of muck. The hose may spray water or light—whatever feels right to you. Dust away the dust or collect the rubbish and throw it in the bin. As the stickiness, dust, or rubbish is removed or washed away, collect it all into the bin.

Move down into your torso, through your arms and legs, and clean away anything that needs cleaning. You may not be able to clean everything out in one session—that's okay.

When the bin is full, put it into the elevator, watch the doors close, and let the bin be taken away. Wait for the elevator doors to open again and step inside. The bin is gone, and you can now press the button to return to the ground floor. When the elevator doors open, open your eyes.

My Experience:

This is a meditation I did several times, and each time I washed more blackness away, revealing a soft, clean pink underneath. I had a large industrial-size bin to begin with, and as I repeated the meditation at different times, I noticed the bin became smaller each time until I was carrying one the size of a wastepaper basket. This was so empowering and cleansing! I go back to it every now and then if I feel some icky energy in my body.

Crisis Support Resources

Information current at time of publishing 2025. These are crisis support resources for Australia only.

AUSTRALIA WIDE
000 – Emergencies only – police, ambulance, fire
Phone 000

1800 RESPECT
National domestic violence support
Phone 1800 737 732, text 0458 737 732
www.1800RESPECT.org.au

Lifeline - Crisis support services
Phone 13 11 14

QLD
DV Connect - Be heard, be safe
Phone 1800 811 811
www.dvconnect.org

SA
24 Hr Domestic Violence Crisis Line
Phone 1800 800 098
Women's Safety Services SA
www.womenssafetyservices.com.au

NT
The Salvation Army NT
Phone (08) 8981 5928
www.salvationarmy.org.au

NTCOSS
Northern Territory Council of Social Services
Phone (Darwin) (08) 8948 2665

NSW
NSW Domestic Violence Line
Phone 1800 65 64 63
www.nsw.gov.au/community-services/domestic-and-family-support

ACT
24/7 ACT crisis line
Phone 02 62 800 900
www.dvcs.org.au

VIC
**Safe Steps Victoria's 24/7
family violence response centre**
Phone 1800 015 188
www.safesteps.org.au

TAS
Safe at Home Tasmania
Phone 1800 608 122
www.safeathome.tas.gov.au

WA
Women's Domestic Violence Helpline
Phone 1800 007 339
Centre for Women's Safety and Wellbeing
https://cwsw.org.au

www.ingramcontent.com/pod-product-compliance
Lightning Source LLC
Chambersburg PA
CBHW071915290426
44110CB00013B/1372